# Psychodynamic Supervision Theory and Practices

This book sets out a new model for psychodynamic supervision, designed around relational psychoanalytic theory and practice. It emphasizes the development of the self of the therapist and working directly with the emergent therapeutic relationship.

Building on Barsness's seminal *Core Competencies of Relational Psychoanalysis* text, this book is grounded in those theoretical competencies. The author offers what he calls the MAMAL method of supervision—(M—muse; A—affect; M—metabolization; A—articulation; and L—learning), a method that privileges (1) affect over cognition, (2) the use of the therapist's subjectivity as the primary portal to the patient's internal and interpersonal world, (3) the immersion of the supervisor's subjectivity in the supervisory process, and (4) viewing the patient as a muse rather than an object of assessment. The MAMAL method approach enriches the supervisory experience and enhances the therapeutic process, fostering a therapeutic climate where both therapist and patient can thrive. It is attention to our own humanity and woundedness that facilitates a deep connection to our patients and animates the progression of the therapeutic process and is at the core of this supervision model.

Drawing on clinical experience, this book is grounded in research and is a readable resource for psychoanalysts, psychotherapists, and mental health professionals, providing a clear guide to a relational model of supervision and a concise understanding of relational theory and practice.

**Dr. Roy E. Barsness** is the Founder and Executive Director of the Contemporary Psychodynamic Institute. He is the author of the text *Core Competencies of Relational Psychoanalysis*, and he has served as Academic Dean and Professor at The Seattle School of Theology and Psychology, Professor and Clinical Director at Seattle Pacific University, and Clinical Associate Professor at the University of Washington, School of Psychiatry.

Here is what graduates of the Certificate Program in Relational Psycho-analysis at the Contemporary Psychodynamic Institute are saying about their experience with the MAMAL method...

"Working with the MAMAL method for case consultation both as a super-visor and a supervisee has revitalized my work as a psychotherapist. The upside-down approach of tending to affect first has been like finding a hidden door into the depths of relational work that was missing from traditional super-visory approaches. Attention to affect and the unconscious, collaborative au-thority, relentless curiosity and emotional risking are the portals into not only deepening my work with clients, but also are growing myself as a person."

**Mandy Casurella**, *Anchorage, AK*

"Learning and practicing this approach has changed the way I work in a way that feels more alive, engaging and deeply beneficial to my patients. Dr. Barsness' and his efforts to scaffold the supervision endeavor in this way is both practical and creative, structured, and endlessly flexible as I learn to use my own humanity in my work with other humans."

**Cristine Ramsdale**, *Seattle, WA*

"I am so deeply grateful that I found this model of supervision early in my career. It requires me as a therapist to acknowledge my own subjectivity and the fact that it is always active in the room as I work with my patients. I haven't stopped practicing this model since I began four years ago, and I can't imagine doing this sort of work without it now."

**Joe Hall**, *Grand Rapids, MI*

"In this groundbreaking book, Dr. Barsness takes us on a revolutionary journey through the world of supervision and consultation. As a psycholo-gist with two decades of experience, I found his method to be transforma-tive, leading to increased self-awareness and enriched patient care. I found myself invigorated and enlightened by Barsness' innovative approach, dis-covering new depths within myself, leading to greater authenticity and openness both personally and professionally. This book not only offers practical techniques but also inspires a profound shift in perspective, ul-timately enriching the therapeutic process for both practitioners and pa-tients alike. Highly recommended for practitioners seeking personal and professional growth."

**Jeremy Morris**, *Salina, KS*

"With five years of work in the MAMAL method of consultation, I now use this model for my training clinic for all clinicians because of its impact on my own clinical work and mind. I find that the model has given us space to move towards a richer, more honest dialogue with one another as clinicians, and more wholehearted authenticity with our clients. Most impactful – for me in my own life, my work as a clinician, and in my therapeutic community at our clinic – is that I have found the model has helped me to hide less, and in that, feel far less alone in my world."

**Jeremy Dew**, *College Station, TX*

"The MAMAL method has helped me increase my understanding of human pains and to heal and grow as a psychotherapist and a person in an experiential, collaborative, supportive, loving, authentic, and relational environment. I gained not only knowledge but also insight and experiences, and I feel more grounded and connected to myself and to my clients at a deeper level."

**Hiromi Gerety**, *Seattle, WA*

"The MAMAL method of supervision has transformed the way I show up in the room with my patients as well as given me deeper access to myself both personally and professionally. This model has helped me to stop hiding behind intellectualizing, theorizing, rigid adherence to modalities, and treating my patients as objects to be fixed. Likewise, it has grown my capacity and ability to locate myself and the courage to show up as fully as possible with my patients creating opportunities for authentic encounters, intersubjectivity, and more life-giving work. My experience is that the more I have learned to show up through these relational encounters, the more the work has moved from 'a grind' to enlivening for all involved."

**Ben Reisterer**, *Grand Rapids, MI*

"This thoughtful and extremely relational model of supervision that Dr. Barsness created and developed has guided my approach from the mindset of needing to know, with little room to be wrong in my work to a beautiful melodic rhythm that combines the notes of my clinical mind, my embodied life experience, and trust in my intuitions and inclinations. This approach has opened space inside me and towards my patients on its emphasis on curiosity, exploration, and creativity. Traditional supervision tends to pay less attention to the affective and intuitive experiences of the therapist, whereas the MAMAL method understands and highlights the therapeutic encounter as an embodied one and as a bridge to the patient's life experiences in ways. Working from this perspective has reshaped me and now guides me as I work with myself in deeper ways and guide others to their own understanding and healing, I highly recommend this book for all of these reasons and many more."

**Marjorie Long**, *Birmingham, AL*

"Experiencing MAMAL alongside other courageous therapists who did not hide behind relational psychoanalytic theory but instead chose to live out this theory together accelerated my growth as a relational psychodynamic therapist far beyond my expectations. As a result of learning how to listen with my full being (not just my mind) I feel much more present and alive both inside and outside the therapy room. I am so thankful for Dr. Barsness' creative mind and work and also for my experience at the *Contemporary Psychodynamic Institute*!"

**Shannon Gilbride**, *Encinitas, CA*

"Experiencing MAMAL alongside other therapists accelerated my growth as a relational psychodynamic therapist. As a result of learning how to listen with my full being (not just my mind) I feel much more present and alive both inside and outside the therapy room. I'm so thankful for Roy's creative mind and work and also CPI!"

"Truly a unique consultation and supervision model that enlivened my own clinical practice and supervision process. Prizing the clinician's affective experience of the client as the window to understanding, this psychodynamic supervision model values authenticity, curiosity, metabolization, courageous speech, and a trust in one's subjectivity. It has changed the way I practice for the better, as a professor the way I teach and as a clinical supervisor the way I supervise!"

**Cayla Bland**, *La Mirada, CA*

"It is no exaggeration for me to say that the MAMAL Method has reinvigorated my work as a psychotherapist and supervisor. Transformation within the context of psychotherapy occurs in relational space between therapist and patient. More than a technique, this model is dedicated to the development of the self of the therapist so that the therapist can show up more fully and courageously as a participant within that relational space. It is a therapeutic model that is both generative and creative in its essence and I would say, is relatively rare! This book is a must read for psychotherapists."

**Bryan Nixon**, *Grand Rapids, MI*

"The MAMAL method truly is an innovative and exciting approach to case consultation where learning and growth come from the inside out and we get to engage and play in the relational realm instead of just talking about the theory and its application. In this book, Dr. Barsness does an excellent job describing the structure and process of running case consult groups using the MAMAL method while also providing the depth of thoughtfulness and purpose behind the creation of this model."

**Clarissa Hill**, *Seattle, WA*

"This model of supervision has had a tremendous impact on me, both professionally and personally. Giving up the need to be the 'Good Enough' object in favor of relating authentically has freed me to live more authentically in my life as well as my work. This model has produced in me confidence in trusting the process and the therapeutic dyad's ability to work intersubjectively including the navigating of conflict towards living with more vitality."

**Ryan Eberst**, *Plano, TX*

"As a psychologist, professor, and clinical supervisor, the MAMAL method has been transformative. Grounded in relational theory and experience, it captures both the heart and mind of psychodynamic supervision with clarity and sophistication. It is essential reading for all clinicians who seek to enhance their therapeutic presence and impact."

**Stanley Hoover**, *Atlanta, GA*

"This supervision model encourages me to access and accept parts of myself that I longed for, but never thought, could be useful in the therapy room. The method not only helps me access those parts of myself but goes further in teaching me HOW to use those parts of myself in a way that is beneficial to the client. My work, and my life, have become enriched, enlivened, and emboldened in ways I always hoped the therapeutic process could entail."

**Chris Roberts**, *Nashville, TN*

"What sets the MAMAL model apart is that it is experiential and affect-focused. Because each person is asked to engage the patient being presented from a relational stance it expands not only the mind of the presenter, but the mind of every therapist in the room. It has transformed the way I consult and do therapy."

**Kelly Garrett**, *Vancouver, WA*

# Psychodynamic Supervision Theory and Practices

In a New Key

**Roy E. Barsness**

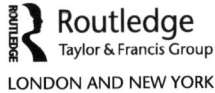
Routledge
Taylor & Francis Group

LONDON AND NEW YORK

Designed cover image: Getty Images © Shaumiaa Vector

First published 2025
by Routledge
4 Park Square, Milton Park, Abingdon, Oxon, OX14 4RN

and by Routledge
605 Third Avenue, New York, NY 10158

*Routledge is an imprint of the Taylor & Francis Group, an informa business*

*British Library Cataloguing-in-Publication Data*
A catalogue record for this book is available from the British Library

*Library of Congress Cataloging-in-Publication Data*
Names: Barsness, Roy E., author.
Title: Psychodynamic supervision theory and practices: in a new key / Roy E. Barsness.
Description: Abingdon, Oxon; New York, NY: Routledge, 2025. |
Includes bibliographical references and index. |
Identifiers: LCCN 2024035846 (print) | LCCN 2024035847 (ebook) |
ISBN 9781032871653 (paperback) | ISBN 9781032874760 (hardback) |
ISBN 9781003532828 (ebook)
Subjects: MESH: Psychotherapy, Psychodynamic--methods | Models, Psychological |
Professional-Patient Relations | Psychoanalytic Theory
Classification: LCC RC480.5 (print) | LCC RC480.5 (ebook) | NLM WM 420.5.P75 |
DDC 616.89/14—dc23/eng/20240912
LC record available at https://lccn.loc.gov/2024035846
LC ebook record available at https://lccn.loc.gov/2024035847

ISBN: 978-1-032-87476-0 (hbk)
ISBN: 978-1-032-87165-3 (pbk)
ISBN: 978-1-003-53282-8 (ebk)

DOI: 10.4324/9781003532828

Typeset in Optima LT Std
by codeMantra

If interested in further training and learning opportunities in Relational Psychodynamic Therapy at the Contemporary Psychodynamic Institute, please follow the link below: www.psychodynamicinstitute.com

To
Bryan, Clarissa, Mandy, Chris and Krista
+
To all the alumni and the current and future participants at the
Contemporary Psychodynamic Institute
With gratitude

# Contents

# Preface

Someone once asked me why we do this for a living, I answered,

*Because to us, to do anything else would not be living.*
*For who else is granted the sacred gift of tending to another person's*
*tattered and broken soul?*
*Who else, is called as witness to discover the depth and beauty of a*
*person,*
*when they or others can no longer see?*
*Who else, is called to listen to all that has been left unsaid, seeking voice?*
*Who else is called to become entangled in the story*
*so that a new story*
*can be written?*
*And who else, discovers their own soul, when they have touched*
*the soul of*
*another?*
*Why do we do this for a living? How can we not?*

# Acknowledgments

In my journey of writing and teaching over the years, it is the collective spirit of inquiry, collaboration, and dedication that transforms the solitary act of writing into a shared endeavor of growth and discovery. Thank you to all who have contributed to this remarkable excursion!

To craft a book is to embark upon an expedition of self-discovery, guided by the muses who inspire our voice. These muses are the catalysts for creativity, igniting a passion that fuels the cycle of writing, rewriting, and revising. They are the champions who spur us on when we falter, embodying the very essence of our drive.

Throughout my career as a professor, clinician, and writer, my students have been my muses, challenging me with their inquiries and pushing me to articulate the intricacies of psychotherapy. They have been the driving force behind my efforts to structure complex theoretical constructs of psychoanalysis, leading to the creation of my first book, *Core Competencies in Relational Psychoanalysis: A Guide to Practice, Study and Research*. This text *Psychodynamic Supervision: A New Approach* is In a New Key provides the foundational elements of practice influenced by those theoretical constructs, presenting a training model for clinical practice.

I am indebted to each student who has taught me, challenged me, and served as muse, allowing me to share my understanding of the therapeutic process. It is my hope that by assembling these insights into one place, these books will continue to foster the growth of theory and practice for all who engage with them.

The publication of the *Core Competencies* text inspired Paul Steinke, then VP of Alumni Relations at the Seattle School where I was a professor, to organize an Alumni Book Tour. The success of this tour revealed a profound desire for post-graduate professional supervision and training, which, in turn, led to the development of a certificate program in relational psychodynamic therapy. I am forever grateful to Paul, personally, and for his foresight, belief, and unwavering support.

In preparation for launching the new certificate program, I selected three former teaching assistants—Clarissa Hill, Bryan Nixon, and Krista Law—and embarked on an intensive training program to prepare them as supervisors/trainers for the certificate program. Their contributions to curriculum development were invaluable, and I am deeply appreciative of the bond we formed.

The first cohort of the program not only graduated but also stayed on becoming the foundational members in the development of the *Contemporary Psychodynamic Institute*. The three-year certificate program in relational psychodynamic therapy is central to the Institute and has evolved into an experiential training platform and a vibrant community of life-long learners. My heartfelt thanks go to Cayla Bland, Mandy Casurella, Jeremy Dew, Ryan Eberst, Jamie Fenimore, Matt Inman, Jessica Miller, and Chris Roberts—whose enthusiasm and dedication to the vision brought the Institute into existence and to Nicole Greenwald for her entrepreneurial savvy and technical knowledge in creating the structure for the new institute.

I would also like to express my gratitude to Clarissa Hill, Mandy Casurella, Chris Roberts, Kirk Webb, Brad Strawn, David Baker, Shannon Gilbride, Lynne Gregory, and Jennifer Jones. Your feedback on the manuscript has been instrumental in enhancing the presentation of this book and provided me with continued encouragement. I am very grateful to the editorial and production team at the Routledge Publishing Company. Thank you to Editor Kate Hawes for her interest in the publication of this text, Assistant Editor Deepika Batra in her shepherding this project through and to the project management team including Project Manager Kishore Sivakolundu, and CodeMantra team. Thank you to all for your patience and guidance in the completion of this text.

With deep gratitude.

# 1 So What's New?

I was three years old when my older brother and his friend convinced me that I could ride a slippery pig named Ziggy, snorting around in its pen. As you can imagine it did not go well. At least for me. For my brother and his friend—well—they laughed their heads off and warned me not to tell our mother. So, it is with psychoanalysis. Trying to corral psychoanalysis is a bit like trying to corral Ziggy. Just as you think you can, you can't. And sometimes when we think we have or that we can—we rope our ideologies into a dogma and proclaim them as truth. Psychoanalysis refuses to be corralled. And that is a very good thing. Psychoanalysis at its core is a deeply human encounter, and each patient and each session are unique. It is a profound emotional, human–human event that is difficult to explain or quantify. Freud (1912) compared psychoanalysis to the game of chess where "only the opening and closing of the game admit of exhaustive systematic description…and that the gap left in between can only be filled in by the zealous study of games fought out by master hands…Given the exceptional diversity in the mental constellations concerned, the plasticity of all mental processes, and the great number of the determining factors involved prevent the formulation of a stereotyped technique." However, he continues, "These circumstances do not prevent us from establishing a procedure for the physician which will be found most generally efficient" (p. 342).

So, in this text and in my text *Core Competencies in Relational Psychoanalysis* (2018), I have essentially been silly enough to do some corralling. Why? I think there are two reasons. The first is, psychoanalysis provides a very rich theory of the mind. But when it comes to a coherent theory of clinical practice it gets a little slippery as it has not clearly explained core clinical practices. In fact, "the issue of technique has often been viewed as, if not exactly a dirty topic, one that is a bit unseemly" and something [Mitchell wryly noted] for "mere technicians, a lesser calling" (Tublin, 2018, p. 68).

From my first encounter with psychoanalysis, I was smitten with the complexity of the theory, terrified that I wasn't fully understanding it, and certainly flummoxed by how to practice it—a common refrain I hear from many. But, just as one is drawn to the aloof amour that one desires so intensely yet is uncertain if one can woo, I dedicated the remainder of my

DOI: 10.4324/9781003532828-1

career to understanding psychoanalytic theory that eventually developed into a schema for clinical practices. Through my studies and research, I discovered a shared structure in which we conduct psychoanalysis, a structure that is not restrictive and, most importantly, recognizes the exceptional diversity within one's own theory and practices as well as the uniqueness of the therapist's personality and their relationship with the patient.

The second reason I ended up developing a structure of psychoanalytic disciplines and a supervision method to develop these disciplines is because, as a life-long professor in psychology graduate programs, I had to develop course descriptions, learning objectives, assignments to meet those objectives, and evaluation grids to determine whether the course objectives had been met. As a result, I had to do some corralling to meet institutional and accrediting body pressures as well as student needs. As students entered their internships and experienced their first exposure to evidenced-based models, which they found more comprehensible, in contrast to the analytic theories they found obscure, inaccessible, and the practice of it "squishy," I felt a call to some action. As one student lamented, "I have all this theory, but I don't know what to do." Consequently, I decided to begin to research common analytic practices and to work more intentionally in translating and communicating rich and complicated psychoanalytic theory into how we practice.

I felt a deep commitment to my students to be able to go out into the clinical world and speak with clarity and confidence about the psychoanalytic techniques they have, just as confidently as those who dominate the field with their manualized, evidence-based treatments.

All of that said, the scaffolding that I have developed through research, my own practices, and years and years of teaching means nothing—unless you the therapist "shows up." It is the therapist's vulnerability and willingness to yield their strongly held insecurities hidden behind their theoretical dogma and surrender to the relational processes between themselves and their patients that define relational psychodynamic therapy (RPT). The MAMAL supervision method (M—muse; A—affect; M—metabolization; A—articulation; and L—learning) is predicated and grounded within this theoretical disposition and forms the supervision model described in this text. It is the attention to our own humanity and woundedness that facilitates a deep connection to the woundedness of our patients, and it is that which animates the progression of the therapeutic process. This central aspect of therapist vulnerability is often considered secondary, if at all, in most supervision models, but is at the core of the MAMAL method. Supervisees actively pursue a radical openness to their own selfhood, attend to and metabolize the affective states occasioned by their patients, and courageously find ways to work authentically with them.

Three decades of research conducted by the Third Interdivisional American Psychological Task Force on Evidenced-Based Relationships and Responsiveness asking the question "What specifically is effective in the powerful psychotherapy relationship?" (Norcross & Lambert, 2018, p. 306) found that "the curative contribution of the person of the therapist is, arguably, as evidence based as are manualized treatments of psychotherapy methods" (Hubble et al., 2011, in Norcross & Lambert, 2018, p. 306). Furthermore, that "multiple and converging sources of evidence indicate that *the person of the psychotherapist is inextricably intertwined with the outcome of psychotherapy* (italics mine)" (Norcross & Lambert, 2018, p. 307), and that "psychotherapy relationships make substantial and consistent contributions to patient outcome independent of specific types of psychological treatment method" (Norcross & Lambert, 2018, p. 308); and *yet* [italics mine] current "treatment guidelines give short shrift—some would say lip service—to the person of the therapist and the emergent therapeutic relationship" (Norcross & Lambert, 2018, p. 307). Therefore, a central goal of RPT is to help develop the self of the therapist.

Bruno Bettelheim (1903–1990), a prominent psychoanalyst born in Freud's hometown of Vienna lived and breathed Freudian thought from his early childhood. In his book, *Freud, and Man's Soul: An Important Re-Interpretation of Freudian Theory* (1982), Bettelheim laments how the English translation makes Freud's "direct and always deeply personal appeals to our common humanity appear to English readers as abstract, depersonalized, highly theoretical, erudite, and mechanized-in short, 'scientific'-statements about the strange and very complex workings of our mind" (p. 5).

He says his students at the University of Chicago, where he was a professor in mid-life, possessed excellent understanding of theory, but their understanding of theory was a "reasoned out, emotionally distant understanding" (Bettelheim, 1982, p. 5). Their detachment bothered Bettelheim, for he says what the patient needs is an "emotional closeness based on an immediate sympathetic comprehension of their soul – of what afflicted it, and why" (Bettelheim, 1982, p. 5). He said Freud believed analysis required a "spontaneous sympathy of our unconscious with that of others, a feeling response of our soul to theirs" (Bettelheim, 1982, p. 7). Bettelheim argues that lost in translation is how important it is for clinicians to take theory personally and to be encouraged to gain access to their own unconscious and to "everything else that is most human" (Bettelheim, 1982, p. 6). Bettelheim found his students had developed a psychoanalytic attitude of "trying to comprehend other people through the spectacle of abstraction…never turning their gaze inward to the soul of their own unconscious." He continues, "…they did not give enough thought to the fact that Freud, in order to create psychoanalysis and the unconscious had to analyze his own dreams, understand his own slips of the tongue and the reason he forgot things or made various other mistakes" (Bettelheim, 1982, p. 7).

In other words, to find the soul of another, one must first look into their own.

If emotional healing of traumas past is the intent of psychotherapy, it would appear we need to turn our eyes inward, to find our patients to be part of their healing process.

The relational psychoanalytic movement emphasizes the vital role of the therapist's self-experience within the therapeutic process where change occurs through the "interpenetration of [two] minds, conscious and unconscious" (Benjamin, 2018, p. 1). This shift demands of us our vulnerability and to continually be developing ourselves as we step out of a stance of objectivity into the space of intersubjective play.

Working within intersubjective play, child psychoanalyst Donald Winnicott also reminds us of the importance of attending to the therapist's own personal experience, exploring these ideas through various essays, such as *The Use of Object Relating through Identifications* (1969) and *Playing and Reality* (1971), suggesting that we must undergo a critical personal experience in order to deeply comprehend our patient. We must have an awareness and acceptance of our own human condition, our strengths, our flaws, our fears, our shame, and frankly, a humility that connects with the challenge of simply being human to understand our patients, and to value the therapist's self-experience as a primary source for change within our patients' lives. The therapist's subjectivity is a critical turn in psychoanalytic theory. This turn shifted our understanding of what constitutes change, namely, that change occurs with two minds (therapist and patient) intersecting, in juxtaposition to one mind (the analyst) abstractly analyzing the mind of another (the patient), requiring greater attention to the self of the therapist in relation to their patient.

And *yet* [italics mine] **as noted above** current "treatment guidelines give short shrift—some would say lip service—to the person of the therapist and the emergent therapeutic relationship" (Norcross & Lambert, 2018, p. 307).

The MAMAL method of supervision seeks to correct this error, with a strong emphasis on the development of the self of the therapist and learning to work directly with the emergent relationship between the therapist and the patient.

Conventional supervisory relationships follow a teaching model, where the clinically advanced supervisor shoulders the responsibility of advising, critiquing, offering feedback, and imparting theoretical and clinical knowledge. These relationships tend to shy away from delving into working with the self of the therapist and the affective states experienced within the therapist occasioned by the patient. Rather the supervisory process tends to lean toward a cognitive assessment of the presented case. Though relational psychoanalytic theory holds to the essential value of the subjectivity of the self, the supervisory endeavor within psychoanalysis also still trends toward a cognitive assessment by focusing on the patient and the supervisor's authority rather than upon co-metabolizing the affective stirrings that emerge within the therapist, the supervisor, and the in-between, elicited in relation to the patient.

Psychoanalyst Jonathan Slavin (1997) says that the analytic supervisor as authority and dispenser of truth has been reluctant to change, referring to "psychoanalytic training programs…as similar to the initiation rites of clerical candidates" [arguing] that a century after its birth, psychoanalysis still is too often taught as truth rather than as possibility. He suggests that, "supervision more akin to Ferenczi's view of co-construction" would grant a much deeper understanding to the analytic and supervisory experience, believing that "mutuality, shared and authorized power and the co-construction of knowledge grants a much deeper understanding of the supervisory process and to the patients with whom they present" (in Frawley-O-Dea & Sarnat, 2000, p. 24). Though relational psychoanalytic theory emphasizes the use of the self of the therapist, working within a collaborated space of intersubjectivity and working through conflict interpersonally, we have yet to develop a relational supervision model.

The MAMAL method discussed in this text seeks to change that by focusing on the self of the therapist and attending to deep affective states and working intersubjectively, I believe accomplishes it. The method privileges (1) affect over cognition, (2) the use of the therapist's subjectivity as the primary portal to the patient's internal and interpersonal world, (3) the immersion of the supervisor's subjectivity in the supervisory process, and (4) a focus on the patient as inspiration rather than as an object to evaluate.

Several years ago, in my supervision practice, I began to feel something was missing. While practicing the typical elements of supervision, such as assessing and thinking about the patient's presentation and suggesting to the therapist what they might do or what I would do to further the clinical experience, I realized we were engaged primarily in an intellectual exercise. The emotions we were experiencing were absent much of the time. I started asking what ultimately has become a fundamental orienting question within the MAMAL method, "What affective states does this patient stir within the self of the therapist (and the supervisor), and how is it informing the therapeutic process?"

I realized that in investigating cases from a purely cognitive, intellectual position, we lost touch with our primary access point to the patient—the therapist's emotional responses and the relational experience within the therapeutic dyad. This realization caused me to shift my focus from concentrating solely on the patient to more fully attending to the affective states being aroused within the therapist in direct relationship to the patient. By focusing on what was happening in the *gut* that is the internal processes occurring within the therapist, a notable contrast emerged between the therapist's actions (e.g., empathic listening, offering insights, interpretation, and advice) and the therapist's underlying. Rarely did they express their experience of the patient or the evolving relationship between them. Yet, probing into "what was going on in their gut/viscera" revealed a profound reservoir of emotion, unexplored intuitions, unconscious urges, and relational tensions, of which the patient was unaware, though most likely sensed and had some conscious or unconscious awareness of. It seemed to me that if the patient did not have full access to our minds and our affects, the therapy was compromised.

My supervisees and I began to recognize that what is being emotionally stimulated within the therapist is, in part, a transmission of the patient's internal and external world, yet unknown or unspoken. Therefore, it became important (urgent) to prioritize listening to the "story that was beyond words" spoken through the affective experiences of the therapist, the patient, and the patient–therapist relationship. When the therapist began articulating their experience to the patient, the treatment enlivened, discovering that holding back affect and interpersonal experiences was detrimental not only to the patient but also to the therapist.

The discovery of the MAMAL method of supervision introduced a new approach that emphasizes the following.

### The Development of the Self of the Therapist

- **Deep Dive into Subjectivity:** The therapist's self is recognized as a crucial element in successful treatment, necessitating a profound exploration of their own subjectivity.

### Primacy of Affect

- **Emotional Responses:** The therapist's emotional responses to the patient are utilized as the primary means of establishing contact with the patient.

### Patient as Muse

- **Clinical Creativity:** The patient is viewed as a source of inspiration for clinical creativity, rather than merely an object for analysis.

### Structured Supervision Process

Each participant uses the presenting case as a Muse and follows these steps:

- **Sharing Affective Reactions:** Participants share the affective states elicited by the patient/Muse.
- **Metabolizing Experiences:** Participants link past and present relationships instrumental in the formation of the patient's life, considering how and why these patterns are demonstrating themselves within the therapist/patient dyad. A guiding question is: "What happened and what is happening?"
- **Practicing Articulation:** Participants practice articulating their thoughts and affective experiences to the patient aloud. This is not a rehearsal for actual patient interactions but a method to intensify and deepen clinical awareness and understanding through vocalization.
- **Engaging in Learning:** Participants consider the theoretical and clinical insights gained, recognizing that learning is an on-going, non-linear process throughout supervision.
- **Vulnerability and Connection:** Emphasizing self-awareness and emotional openness, the MAMAL model nurtures vulnerability, which in turn

cultivates profound connections within the group. These bonds often evolve into lasting relationships that are integral to the therapist's professional development and support network.

No two therapists work in the same fashion and given the uniqueness of each relationship and the working through of what happens in that relationship, it must be so. However, a supervision model that holds to the primacy of affect; the use of the therapist's self and a supervisor embedded within the process where the patient serves as muse for co-metabolization, vitalizes the clinicians work, while respecting their distinctiveness. The structure that the MAMAL method claims authority about process (structure) alongside a radical openness to that which emerges and unfolds within the therapeutic process. Nancy McWilliams' (2018) analogy of the analyst as "trailblazer" is helpful. She states, "if one is in an alien jungle, one needs to be with someone who knows how to traverse that terrain without encountering danger or going around in circles. The guide does not need to know where the parties will emerge from the wilderness but does have the knowledge to make the journey safe" (in Barsness, 2018, p. 90).

I began this chapter speaking of the need for structure, but also with a concern that structure is second in command to the interpersonal connection between the self of the therapist and the patient, and that the primary "technique" in relational psychodynamic work is the self of the therapist. It is the attention to our own humanity and woundedness that facilitates a deep connection to the woundedness of our patients and it is that which stimulates the progression of the therapeutic process.

With that in mind, I wish to end this chapter with a story my good friend David Baker (2004) tells of an early experience in his life when he was living in Africa. David writes,

In 1983 I was twenty-four years old and in my fifth month of what would be a two-year frolic in Zaire, Africa, now the Democratic Republic of the Congo. I took several jobs, one of which was working for an NGO as a driver shuttling American college students to remote outposts along the Congo River to participate in summer service projects. One hot summer morning I was assigned to drive twelve students to several remote villages along the eastern edge of that great river. Using machetes to open a thin road through the dense jungle, we drove for six bone-crushing hours over rock, through sand and mud, and finally arrived in one of the river villages early in the evening. We planned to stay the night and depart the following morning for our final destination, a village further upriver. The Chief of this village was an engaging man with three wives, many children, likely in his eighties. As night fell, we sat around a fire and, with the help of a translator, talked into the night, his Lingala meeting my English. I and several intrepid students engaged the Chief in an animated conversation that lasted long into the morning hours. Topics varied, from cooking to politics, and as the night progressed the students turned to their huts.

The Chief and I and two women remained, one of whom who was a wife, the other a translator from Kinshasa who doubled as our cook. We sat on wood stumps next to a fire and were soothed by the drums played by young men on the outskirts of the village. Their rhythms ascended and descended through the forest like an audible smoke, finally reaching our ears, lulling us further into even more spirited conversation. The conversation turned particularly passionate as the Chief began to describe the mystic visions and theological perspectives of his tribe, a Bantu group that had absorbed hundreds of years of spiritual stories rooted in the common animism of the Central African culture.

Having just completed an undergraduate degree in theology and planning to return to seminary after Africa, I brought a full head of theological steam to the dialogue, along with a head full of myself. I engaged the Chief, questioning why, and how and if. How could he believe such things, such mystical, earthy, unscientific, and, worst of all, unorthodox ideas? But the Chief's fierce gentility and passionate certainty conveyed a depth of experience of the transcendent that I'd not encountered in my own faith. After I explained in detail some of the major tenets of Christianity—the Trinitarian nature of God, the deity of Christ, the inspiration of the Scriptures—he looked at the ground, and after a long pause leaned forward and whispered to the translator a short sentence, the weight of which stunned me then, and shakes me now in the retelling. It also distilled for me the entire essence of the on-going debate between intellect and experience. The translator leaned toward me and said, "This Chief say, 'The difference between your religion and ours is that you believe your religion; we dance ours." At that, the Chief rose to his feet and began to circle the fire in fluid movements, arms waving, hopping on one foot, chanting and singing. I wish I'd thought to ask the translator the words to the song he sang. But I was mentally numbed, shaken by his words and the dancing gestures that seemed to embody them. I was thrown off balance by their simplicity, feeling the depth of his experience of his own faith, faith as dance, as the present moment, as embodied existence. In those moments, I remember imagining God looking down on us both, and wondering what she must have been thinking.

In reflection, years later, I like to think I can guess: God wasn't thinking at all; God was dancing. And now, in mid-life, after a dozen bouts of belief and disbelief, I am slowly choosing to believe again, but in a different God now—the only God worth believing in—is a Dancing God.

## Who Is This Book for?

Following the publication of the text *Core Competencies in Relational Psychoanalysis: A Guide to Practice, Study and Research*, I discovered a strong desire for further teaching and supervision while providing workshops and seminars on the new text. These requests inspired me to develop a three-year Certificate Program in Relational Psychodynamic Therapy at the Contemporary Psychodynamic Institute. The students and alumni in the certificate program have served as my *muse* for this book, and every word bears their imprint. Therefore, this book is devoted to them and to their continued growth and learning.

This book is also for supervisors interested in a new approach to supervision from a relational psychodynamic model.

Grounded in relational psychodynamic theory and practice, it is a valuable, readable resource for anyone interested in relational psychodynamic theory, whether they supervise it or not.

Lastly, this book can be useful for supervisors and educators in graduate and post-graduate level institutions from other modalities interested in a new way of conducting supervision. Though this supervision model focuses on the development of relational psychodynamic principles, the uniqueness of the MAMAL method lies in its applicability to any mode of treatment. It will be particularly useful in group practicum and case conference situations.

Now let's go dance.

## References

Baker, D. (2024). Personal communication.

Benjamin, J. (2018). *Beyond doer and done to: Recognition theory, intersubjectivity and the third*. New York: Routledge.

Bettelheim, B. (1982). *Freud, and man's soul: An important re-interpretation of Freudian Theory*. New York: Vintage Books.

Frawley-O-Dea, G., & Sarnat, J. (2000). *The supervisory relationship: A contemporary psychodynamic approach*. New York: Guildford Press.

McWilliams, N. (2018). Core competency Two: Therapeutic Stance/Attitude. In R. E. Barsness, (Ed.), *Core competencies in relational psychoanalysis* (Chapter 5). London. Routledge.

Norcross, J. C., & Lambert, L. (2018). Psychotherapy relationships that work III. *Psychotherapy, 55*(4), 303–315.

Slavin, J. (1997). The analytic supervisor as authority: Reluctance to change. In Frawley-O'Dea, M. G., & Sarnat, J. E. (Eds.), *Advances in supervision: Theoretical and practical perspectives* (pp. 24-36). NY. Guilford Press.

Tublin, S. (2018). Core competency one: Therapeutic intent. In R. E. Barsness, (Ed.), *Core competencies in relational psychoanalysis* (Chapter 4). London. Routledge.

Winnicott, D. W. (1969). The use of an object and relating through identifications. *International Journal of Psychoanalysis, 50*, 711–716.

Winnicott, D. W. (1971). *Playing and reality*. London: Tavistock Publications.

# 2 Theoretical Foundations of Relational Psychodynamic Therapy

As a graduate student many years ago, I recall watching the Gloria tapes of Fritz Perl's (Gestalt Therapy), Albert Ellis' (Rational-Emotive Therapy), and Carl Rogers' (Client Centered Therapy)—three therapeutic movements originating out of psychoanalysis, all three attempting to break the mold of the blank screen analyst. But what they did not break was the authority of the therapist. Most strikingly, even the therapeutic stance of Carl Rogers, who to this day sustains a reputation of empathy and kindness, considered the therapist to essentially be an impersonal participant in the therapy process. Rogers says:

> it is surprising how frequently the client uses the word 'impersonal;' in describing the therapeutic relationship after the conclusion of therapy. This is obviously not intended to mean that the relationship- was cold or disinterested. It appears to be the client's attempt to describe this unique experience in which the person of the counselor-the counselor as an evaluating, reacting person with needs of his own-is so clearly absent. In this sense it is "I,"-personal…the whole relationship is composed of the self of the client, the counselor being depersonalized for the purposes of therapy into being the 'the client's other self.
>
> (p. 208)

Nancy McWilliams (2016) speaks of psychoanalysis as well as most western psychotherapies tending "towards the importance of the neutral, non-disclosing analyst or the client-centered therapies, such as reflective listening, reframing, advising, that deemphasize the importance of the self of the therapist (subjectivity) as a primary activating force in assisting our patients in their mental health. Both modalities issue a warning against the dangers of countertransference. This client-centered focus emerges out of our positivistic, scientist view that places value on objectivity and certainty as the guarantor of competence, validity" (p. 183).

In contrast the relational psychoanalytic movement emphasizes the vital role of the therapist's self-experience within the therapeutic process. This shift acknowledges the interplay of the mind and affective experiences of both the patient and the therapist, where change occurs through the intersection of

DOI: 10.4324/9781003532828-2

two minds. This shift encourages therapists to consider how their subjectivity interpenetrates with their patient's subjectivity, fostering continuous development and clinical wisdom. Vulnerability and self-awareness become essential for a therapist to deeply comprehend the patient's psychic reality. Jessica Benjamin (2018) describes this psychic process in terms of "the interpenetration of [two] minds, conscious and unconscious" (p. 1). This shift sparks in us as clinicians to consider how our subjectivity interpenetrates with our patient's subjectivity and to continually be developing ourselves and our clinical wisdom, as we step out of a stance of objective knowing and into the space of intersubjective.

Relational psychodynamic therapy (RPT), an evidence-based psychotherapy model, understands psychic change through meaningful interactions with one another (Cornelius, 2018; Norcross & Lambert 2018). The Relational Psychodynamic model holds to an understanding that we are conceived in relationship, formed in relationship, harmed in relationship, and transformed through relationship. RPT is grounded in depth psychology, particularly contemporary relational psychoanalysis, interpersonal neurobiology, the dialogical philosophy of Martin Buber, and the presence of the sacred within the therapeutic act. I will discuss each of these below.

## Theoretical Foundation One: Relational Psychoanalysis

Relational psychoanalysis is as much a meta-theory or method that evolves from a wide range of psychoanalytic ideas/theories while offering structure and flexibility in therapeutic practices. In this chapter, I outline the basic theory foundational to relational psychoanalysis and, in Chapters 3 and 5, to relational psychodynamic practices. The practices are based on a qualitative research study (Barsness, 2018) that resulted in seven core disciplines: (1) therapeutic intent, (2) therapeutic stance/attitude, (3) deep listening/affective attunement, (4) the there and then and the here and now, (5) patterning and linking, (6) repetition and working through, and (7) courageous speech disciplined spontaneity—representative of common practices in conducting a relational psychodynamic treatment.

Relational psychoanalysis is a movement that began in the 1980s. At that time, a group of psychoanalysts from the NYU Postdoctoral Program in Psychotherapy and Psychoanalysis (Lew Aron, Neil Altman, Anthony Bass, Jessica Benjamin, Phillip Bromberg, Jody Messler-Davies, Muriel Dimen, Emmanuel Ghent, and Adrienne Harris), influenced by the postmodern movement flourishing at the time, began to rethink historical psychoanalytic theory and practices. The postmodern movement, at its nexus philosophically, psychologically, and culturally, was questioning the norms of the day that prized and emphasized concreteness, certainty, authority, knowledge, rationalism, objectivism, white male supremacy, and heterodoxy. In contrast, those engaged in the postmodern movement began to view life and the human condition from a more subjective view embracing complexity and multiplicity. Born out of this heady philosophical shift at the time, this innovative group of progressive psychoanalytic thinkers ignited a psychoanalytic movement aligned with the emerging philosophy of the postmodern era. The first text of the movement, *Object Relations in Psychoanalytic Theory*, written by Stephen Mitchell and Jay Greenberg in 1983, and their launching of the journal *Psychoanalytic Dialogues* mainstreamed relational psychoanalysis, securing its place within psychoanalytic discourse.

These pioneers introduced a "radical alternative" to the one-person drive theory posited by earlier theoreticians such as Freud, Klein, Winnicott, Kernberg, and Kohut. They advocated for a two-person psychology that emphasized the dyadic, dynamic flow within the therapeutic relationship. Founding member Adrienne Harris states, "The two-person psychologies are perhaps the most dramatic concept that inaugurated the relational turn" (Barsness, 2018, p. 46).

What does a two-person psychology involve? (1) A two-person psychology de-emphasizes the drive model "in which the mind is envisioned as built out of sexual and aggressive impulses and their derivatives to a relational model in which the mind is envisioned out of interactional configurations of self in relation to others" (Mitchell, 1993, p. 9). It is in the interplay of the mind and affective experiences of the patient, and the mind and affective experiences of the therapist, and the interplay of the two where change is made possible. (2) The treatment moves beyond one person analyzing and interpreting the other to greater attention to that which is being repeated in the in-between. The interaction within the dyad becomes the primary therapeutic focus of treatment. (3) The understanding of conflict moves beyond intrapsychic conflict with an enlarged focus on interpersonal conflict. Therefore, more is expected of the therapist as they move from empathy toward authenticity, engage in conflict as dialogue, and collaborate directly with the patient in the enactments, considering their own contribution and what is being repeated between the patient and the therapist. (4) A basic premise of mental processes within a two-person psychology is that a person needs another person's mind in order to understand their own. Therefore, the expression of the therapist's experience of the patient, as well as the expression of the patient's experience of the therapist, is considered relevant and important "grist for the mill."

### Primary Themes of Relational Psychoanalysis

#### Intersubjectivity

This radical two-person alternative introduced the concept of *intersubjectivity* understanding the therapeutic relationship as two minds interpenetrating the other. Founder Stephen Mitchell (1993) states:

> The human psyche, in my view, is both intrapsychic and interpersonal, simultaneously, both a one-person and a two-person phenomenon. The intrapsychic and the interpersonal are perpetually interpenetrating

realms that continually fold into each other...the process of self-discovery generally leads to the discovery of past relationships, and in encountering others, one frequently discovers oneself.

(p. 143)

With the understanding that humans are shaped interpersonally, and that psychopathology is characterized by maladaptive relational configurations, fundamental to relational psychoanalysis is the power of working intersubjectively—that is, directly within the experience of the therapist/patient relationship. Relational psychoanalysts' basic premise is that human beings are born with a primary need of relatedness and that relatedness is necessary for survival and is the primary organizer of mental life.

RPT is built upon a social constructivist paradigm where knowing is socially co-constructed, and emotional processing leads toward cognitive reflection. It is non-binary, dialectical, complex, and perspectival, and growth occurs through conflicting ideals and collaborative authority.

Historically, the therapist's subjectivity (or the therapist's experiencing self) was considered as countertransference. Intersubjectivity, on the other hand, situates insight and the growth of two minds interacting within the rich and complex field of mutuality and bi-directionality. The self is always defining and understanding one's subjectivity in relationship to another self/subject. Thus, the therapist's experience of the patient *and* the patient's experience of the therapist is seen as representative of interdependent interactions that have formed and inform one's understanding of who they are. Working intersubjectively prioritizes interpersonal process over content, affect over cognition, and facilitation of the relational dyad over authoritarianism.

In relational psychoanalysis, transference and countertransference are now reconfigured and understood through an intersubjective lens and the use of our countertransference experiences as passage to a deeper understanding of the patient's internal and interpersonal world. With that in mind, the following excerpt by Barsness and Strawn (2018) in the text *Core Competencies in Relational Psychoanalysis: A Guide to Practice, Study and Research* reads:

> We concur with Donna Orange (1995) who wonders if the use of the word countertransference should be dropped all together, and instead refer to the therapist's and the patient's emotional reactions as co-transference. Gabbard (1996) has stated, "it is generally more clinically useful to consider transference and countertransference as a unit... a joint creation involving contributions from both patient and analyst" (p. 260). In agreement with these theorists, we contend that transference-countertransference theory be repositioned from either/or and be replaced with concepts such as "transferential experience" (Fosshage, 2000), "intersubjectivity" (Atwood, Brandchaft & Stolorow, 1987) or the "interpersonal" (Mitchell, 1988). Transference-countertransference is then essentially perceived as an organism, as transactional,

interactive, and perspectival; a relationship in which there is a "mutual, bi-directional, interactive influence" (Fosshage, 2000, p. 25). In this connection, past, present, and future collide and require the analytic couple to make meaning of all aspects of a person's life as it now presents itself between the two, rather than the one. This complex human encounter gets at the matter of the self-in-relation in an experiential visceral way and moves the patient beyond an isolated, analyzed review of their past. The relational stance challenges a treatment where patients historically were, "shadow companions, ostensibly invited on a mutually intimate journey, but traveling a course piloted by the analyst... [resulting] in an experience in aloneness, a tutorial in free association, replete with intellectual understanding of genetics and dynamics... sprinkled with interpretations that locate pathology within the patient".

(Geist, 2009, p. 66)

The outcome of such an analysis, Barsness and Strawn (2018) continue, "is that the patient ended up with better explanations, but not a better life. What occurs in a relational analysis, however, is not just a good interpretation of the past, but a working through of the interactional conflict, staged and co-produced between both actors—therapist and patient—leading to a more meaningful interpersonal life. In this kind of analysis, we no longer hold to a benign neutrality or hold to the belief that we, as the therapist, are the authority; rather, we are engaged in an intense intimate act of human relations. Intersubjectivity, then, is the intersection of two subjects, two minds, two physical beings, two affective states and working within the complexity of each subject, as it intersects and influences the other" (p. 185).

Intersubjectivity within the therapeutic relationship is extremely complex and can be misunderstood and misused. We understand that the patient-subject is not in our offices to analyze us, while at the same time recognize that in their experience of us, they too are analyzing our moods, shifts, words, and how it feels to be in our presence.

*Intersubjectivity and Countertransference Dominance*

Finnell (1985, as cited in Maroda, 2004) states that "The analytic situation offers much gratification for analysts with intense needs to be loved, idealized, and to feel a sense of power and control over others" (p. 59).

Karen Maroda's (2004) pioneering work on countertransference dominance states that "most instances of countertransference dominance are stimulated or provoked by a need to preserve the therapist's narcissism and block negative transference" (p. 59). Finnel (1985, as quoted in Maroda, 2004,) who says:

.... The analytic situation offers much gratification for analysts with intense needs to be loved, idealized, and to feel a sense of power and control over others. Analysts with such dynamics will tend to promote

idealization, power, and control by taking a dominant position in relation to the analysand who is essentially submissive and masochistic in
these dynamics.... The narcissistic character structure of both is protected, and both receive a great deal of gratification that leaves the basic
pathology untouched.

(p.59)

Maroda advocates that countertransference reactions need to be expressed
and the only way through is by letting the patient in on what has been and is
happening (Maroda, 2004, p. 52). Acting out countertransference reactions
through withdrawal or through narcissistic gratification is disrupted if the
therapist can gain a perspective on what they are doing and why—and have
the courage to communicate this affectively to the patient. When the therapist
authentically engages the patient through personal and affective communication about their countertransference experiences, the countertransference
experience is again made useful and advances the therapeutic process.

As the therapist's own subjectivity is aroused in relationship to the patient's subjectivity, unworked issues within the therapist's own narrative are
frequently awakened. When this occurs, the most common reactions are to
withdraw from the patient, blame the patient, default to advising, or overwhelm the patient with self-disclosure. Given these major pitfalls, it may
seem wise to return to keeping the therapist's experience out of the consulting room. However, this is impossible. From the very first encounter, an interpenetration of two minds and emotional responses begins. I have found that
when I avoid working with my own mind and affective responses, I shut down
because of a negative affective state, which is when I am in most danger of
harming the patient. In contrast, if I attune to the intersubjective movements
and am open to the affective experiences generated within the intersubjective space, there is less risk of dominating the space with my subjectivity (see
Radical Openness, Chapter 5).

But what happens when our countertransference experiences overwhelm
us, and we begin to repeat our traumas onto the patient and use the relationship "for the purpose of attempting to heal ourselves" (Maroda, 2004, p. 49),
or if I intrude my own presence upon my patient by "impinging my subjectivity unbidden by the patient, the part of me that needed to 'analyze,' 'have
good analytic sessions,' to be a 'subject' in an 'intersubjective relationship'
and to 'resolve enactments'" (Grossmark, 2018, p. 27).

In considering our countertransference experiences, rather than deny them
or attempt to place them outside of the realm of what is happening between
the patient and the therapist, I turn to Steven Kuchuck's (2021) reflections on
silent disclosure that are instructive in working through countertransference
reactions. He says, through the "mere act of contemplating" (p. 49) we:

connect or return...to otherwise non-conscious, possibly dissociated, content that the therapist needs access to in order to more fully

understand what he or she is feeling. Related and, as mentioned, si-lent-disclosures [contemplations] carry the potential to help the analyst more closely track the impact of their subjectivity...and represents a middle-ground between the therapist's potentially less impinging exam-ination and use of her subjectivity; on the one hand, and the aforemen-tioned more expressive, possibly therapeutic but potentially obtrusive action of deliberate disclosure.

(pp. 51–53)

I recall a patient who said to me, "I like it when you stop and say, 'I have got to think about this.'" In my silence, I was trying to locate myself, get a feel for my subjective experience with my patient before I could bring it into the space for us to both play with. If the therapist can remain open to their subjective uprisings and is able to hold to their subjectivity with a stance of contempla-tion, personal and dyadic inquiry, collaboration, and working through, the use of their countertransference reactions is made useful.

### Intersubjectivity and the Regressed Patient

The use of the therapist's subjectivity with regressed patients is often discour-aged. It is thought that due to the trauma of their experience, they do not have the capacity to hold complex affective states or relational nuances. Conse-quently, they are prone to binaries and splits, are unable to self-reflect and symbolize, and are considered compromised in their ability to work inter-subjectively. Though that may be true, it is also true these patients have a unique ability to call out incongruities within the emotional and relational field of the therapist/patient encounter. When these incongruities are denied or explained away, further splitting occurs. Consequently, what every patient requires, including the regressed, is the therapist's authenticity of their felt experience to confirm and verify the patient's own.

Stephen Mitchell (1993) challenges us to think of regression beyond a re-turn to more primitive states. He suggests that to consider the regressed self as the core of the self is too simplistic. The self is far more complicated than that. Is it only the regressed undeveloped self that will get at the heart of the mat-ter with our patients? Or does it also involve their tenacity, recognizing what they have overcome? Mitchell asks us to consider regression as constructive disintegration, where the "contours of the self become less guarded...where regression is not a return...as much as it is a reclaiming of lost potentials, not a retreat but an expansion" (p. 142).

I think we have jumped too quickly into assuming we know patient readi-ness more than they do, and that the regressed patient cannot bear our expe-rience of them. I think this concern can be mitigated by reminding ourselves that it is always our task to pay attention to and work with deep affective states with all patients, regardless of the level of pathology and where timing is co-constructed. Maroda (2004) answers the question, "How will you know what to say and when to say it?" is, "Ask the patient" (p. 87).

Whether a patient is psychologically sophisticated, capable of meaning-making, and possesses the skills for self-reflection, it is the task of the therapist to adjust, merge, and join with the affective state of the patient. As a result, our therapies will be different with each patient given the level of relational trauma the patient has experienced, as well as the coping mechanisms they have constructed. But if we hold to the rule of affect first and tune our ear to what the patient is trying to *show us*, this should guide us as to how the intersubjective space will be piloted. The emphasis in relational work is "withness." The treatment is less about words and more about the patients' felt sense of how they have been received and acknowledged and how successfully they have wrestled with their trauma in this new relationship. Entrance into intersubjective space involves attending to the patient's *and* the therapist's subjective experience: living "within" the unfolding narrative between the therapist and the patient, attending to process over content, affect over cognition, surrender over authoritarianism, inquiry over declaration, and co-metabolization over interpretation. It is this stance that directs us in our interventions. I think a more important question to ask is not if the patient is ready, but if the therapist is. At issue is not what the patient can or cannot bear, but what the therapist can bear.

### Are We Always in an Intersubjective Reverie?

Yes and no. When two people gather, the potential for intersubjective experiences is potentialized. However, it is also true that two people can simply meet and use the other as an object. In fact, this is the most common way in which we interact with one another.

Reflecting on Martin Buber's philosophy, the "I" only exists in relation to another, so in that case, yes, everything is subjective. However, Buber also spoke of the commonness of I-It relations and that I-it and I-Thou relations exist on a continuum. Both modes are necessary in describing our relational existence. I-It relations is the place where we link, categorize, evaluate, metabolize, sort and organize our thoughts about the relational encounter. Buber puts it this way: "in I-It relations," the other is objectified and reduced to the observer's own experience. In I-thou relationships, the other is invited to meet me where I stand, in open, mutual reciprocity. Both modes of speaking are necessary. While our lives in the world benefit in practical ways because of I-It relations, developing personal wholeness requires I-Thou relationships (Buber, M. in Kramer, K. 2003, p. 16). In I-It relations, we remain outside of relationship, where relationship is defined as transactional. The I-It typically involves adjudication, justifications, evaluations, and classifications. In contrast, an I-Thou stance *turns* toward the other as subject rather than object, positioning oneself toward the other directly, uniquely, and surrendering to the discovery of the other.

### The Unconscious

The unconscious can best be described as the storage unit of repressed, unprocessed thoughts and feelings. Fundamental to the practice of psychoanalysis is that the unconscious becomes conscious and available for mentalization and relief. Freud referred to the unconscious as a cauldron of primitive wishes, impulses, and desires that have been repressed. These wishes and impulses are experienced as painful breaks in relating and split off from the conscious mind. Though the unconscious houses negative aggressive and sexual thoughts and desires, it is also considered as a place of creativity—a creativity, however, that fears honest expression. The unconscious is formed within the relational milieu of early object relations and subsequent relational traumas and experiences where relational failure has occurred and where the fear of replication abides.

Current research in interpersonal neurobiology suggests that access to the unconscious has shifted away from cognitive reformulations and is primarily made available through the activation of emotional processes (Schore, 2018). The unconscious must be felt rather than thought. Therefore, to gain access to the unconscious and the obstructive defensive structures that protect it, the psychodynamic therapist turns their attention toward activation of emotional processes. Christopher Bollas (2017) asserts that the development of the self is established prior to thought or language and that "the experience of the object precedes the knowing of it" (p. 89). It is what we "know" but cannot put into words. He refers to this as the "unthought known," a thought that has been felt and experienced but has yet to be reflected upon and integrated. In very general terms, it is something we "know" but cannot bear. Therapy hopes to recapture what a patient knows but cannot bear. Relational psychodynamic theory holds to the idea that the patient knows themselves best—they just don't know that they know—and that it is the task of the therapist to facilitate for and with the patient, what the patient already knows, but has yet to have given it voice.

### Primitive Mental States

Primitive mental states, simply stated, are pre-verbal and unsymbolized; they have yet to be thought or mentalized and lack the capacity for reflection. These states are bodily, unconscious, and affectively held. They arise from the fragility of the human condition, characterized by the simultaneous urge to merge and to separate. We yearn for connection, love, and the embrace of others, yet we also grapple with the terror of annihilation, separation, and misrecognition. This existential fear, encompassing both the fear of death (death instinct) and the fear of life (eros) often leads to dissociation, dysregulation, pain, rage, and terror. Within a two-person psychology, primitive mental states are viewed from an intrapsychic and interpersonal perspective.

First, mental states exist on a spectrum, ranging from the primitive, where the mind cannot symbolize or reflect, to a more mature state capable of organizing thoughts, regulating affect, and engaging in internal dialogue among multiple self-states. However, even in a mature mind, the capacity for primitive self-states persists. We all experience moments of sensory loss and regression into primitive affective state and acknowledge the coexistence of multiple modes of experience as essential to stable functioning.

While many theorists view primitive mental states as pathological (e.g., Klein, Bion, Winnicott), others prefer to see them as inherent aspects of all individuals (e.g., Mitchell, Aron). Recognizing that individuals may become "stuck" in primitive mental states, as evidenced by a compromised capacity for mentalization, it is important to recognize that dissociation of primitive states is not exclusive to patients; therapists may also experience this phenomenon.

This awareness is significant because it shifts our focus away from analyzing the patient's mental structure and toward understanding how these structures manifest affectively in the therapeutic relationship. Adopting this stance, we inevitably find ourselves challenged and provoked, as our own psyches encounter the primitive states of our patients. Our expertise lies in accepting this reality, acknowledging the activation of our own primitive states, and navigating the therapeutic process with vigilance and insight. Through theoretical frameworks such as the two-person psychology and concept of the Third, we endeavor to gather our minds amidst affective arousal, leaning into symbolization and mentalization as we navigate the therapeutic journey together.

### Multiple Self-Theory

Multiple self-theory views the self as complex, non-singular, continuous, and discontinuous. Toni Morrison, in her novel *The Song of Solomon* (2019), captures this theory poetically:

> You think dark is just one color, but it ain't. There are five or six kinds of black. Some silky, some woolly. Some just empty. Some like fingers. And it don't stay still. It moves and changes from one kind of black to another. Saying something is pitch black is like saying something is green. What kind of green? Green like my bottles? Green like a grasshopper? Green like a cucumber, lettuce, or green like the sky is just before it breaks loose to storm? Well, night black is the same way. May as well be a rainbow.
>
> (p. 41)

Rather than thinking of a true self/false self, a phrase most often attributed to psychoanalyst Donald Winnicott (but generally misrepresented), multiple self-theory views the self as a conglomerate of multiple self-states. Though

Winnicott's true self/false self is often considered as binary, his description of the true self defies such an assigned meaning. His description of a true self is a self fully alive, spontaneous and non-defensive, a complex self capable of multiple self-states.

Multiple self-theory can be confused with fragmentation. A fragmented self refers to a person who experiences a multiplicity of self-states but lacks cohesion, dissociates, and does not possess the capacity for differentiation and reflection. Multiple self-theory, on the other hand, implies that the self is comprised of many and varied self-states that are interconnected and cohered through continuity, constancy, and integration. Philip Bromberg beautifully writes:

"Health is the ability to stand in the spaces between realities without losing any of them—the capacity to feel like one self while being many" (Bromberg, 1993, p. 166).

Buber's concept of receiving oneself refers to the capacity to experience the self in the moment, as well as bring forth aspects of the self that have been set aside, a fluid and dynamic self that receives the often rich but conflicting self-states, without fragmentation.

### Conflict Model

When working with two subjectivities interpenetrating the other, collisions, interlocks, impasses, and enactments are seen as inevitable and essential to the process. Growth is achieved when the therapeutic dyad can gain a greater capacity for reflection and to recognize the other as their own separate subject. At the core of any good model or method is an understanding of the nature, purpose, and impact of conflict. We are naturally prone to binary thinking and to seek safety from difference. Conflict is fundamental to who we are, automatically defending ourselves against what we fear. Conflict demonstrates itself in power struggles and is experienced by a lack of recognition of the other's values, culture, and status.

Conflict in psychoanalysis has its origins in the Freudian structural model, where the biological demands of the id-ego-superego seek to find resolve. Interpretation of the conflict between these three states of self was what shaped the analysis. Cure came through insight into these psychic forces and the growing capacity of the ego to hold the tension between primitive id impulses and superego demands. The goal of psychotherapy was to ensure that id impulses were expressed in socially acceptable ways.

In the generation after Freud, Melanie Klein, the progenitor of Object Relations theory along with Fairbairn and Winnicott, placed less emphasis on biological drive theory, positing that we have a fundamental drive toward relationship and, in particular, the mother and her capacity to receive and bear the infant's aggressive and libidinal urges/projections.

Splitting is central to Klein's theory. She held that the baby internalizes or introjects the mother's breast (caregiving) and seeks to unconsciously maintain Good Breast experiences (life instinct). In the child's effort to sustain good object relations, the child seeks to propel or project Bad Breast experiences (hate and aggression—the death instinct). Klein perceived destructiveness (death instinct) within the mother-child dyad through the lens of envy: that mother possesses something the baby does not have. Through the act of projection, the baby rids themselves of their hate. It is through the interpretation of these distorted intrapsychic images/representations that projections are modified and introjected into gratitude, where the mother exists not only for gratification but also is received as a whole person (whole object relations). This transition from what Klein referred to as the paranoid-schizoid position (part objects) to the depressive position (reality) grounds mental stability and increases the capacity for the maintenance of healthy interpersonal relations.

Wilfred Bion who received his training analysis from Melanie Klein took a different track, viewing projection as a means of communication. He viewed projection as the effort to influence the receiver and in turn be influenced by the receiver. It is the bi-directionality of projection that is more aligned with psychodynamic theory. In the relational psychodynamic models, projection and projective identification are viewed through the lens of intersubjectivity and to complementarity and enactment, "where patient and analyst join together, unconsciously, to mutually generate past conflicts that have become uniquely alive in the present" (Maroda, 2018, p. 165). Working through these conflicts results in the patient's increased ability to incorporate, complexify, and symbolize.

Winnicott's (1971) object relational model placed less emphasis on the destructive impulses of the baby evident in Klein's model. He perceived internal conflict as the result of a failed holding environment. He suggested that healthy development is predicated on "good enough mothering" (p. 113), suggesting that emotional problems were the result of a deprivation in "holding" (p. 148).

In Kohut's self-psychology model, deficits in primary caregiving, such as lack of empathy and mirroring, impacted developmental maturation. However, Kohut also further shifted away from internal drives and parental shortcomings, placing a greater emphasis on the environment.

These post-Freudian models and their defection from the instinct drive model focused on the therapist's capacity for containment, empathy, affective attunement, rupture, and repair. Building upon, and in contrast to, these biological and developmental models, psychodynamic theory views psychic conflict *interpersonally* between significant (m)others as much or more so than differentiated mental structures (i.e., Freud's id-ego-superego), Klein's paranoid-schizoid/depressive positions, or through deficits in empathic failure (e.g., Winnicott and Kohut).

The relational-conflict model builds upon early object relations theory, sharing in the understanding that early caregiver figures are responsible for seriously distorting subsequent relatedness. It differentiates itself, however, believing that this distortion is less related to arrested development than it is to, "setting in motion a complex process through which a child builds an interpersonal world" (Mitchell, 1984, p. 476). Conflict, from this viewpoint, is understood not only as deficit in early object relations but also as a result of one's complex relational environment. Powerful life forces, such as sex and aggression, considered relationally, are the effort to make relational contact. When relational efforts for contact are frustrated, unmet, or unseen, the result is disturbances in the mind, body, and spirit. In RPT, treatment moves beyond interpretation, empathy, good-enough mothering, or mirroring. The therapist is now considered to be a part of the patient's complex relational system, and the therapy shifts from observation to *engaging* intrapsychic and interpersonal dramas that are alive historically in the in-between of the therapeutic dyad. Deconstructing and interpreting historical conflict is less threatening than engaging in direct relational conflict with the patient. But it is in the inevitability of *complementarity* and *enactments* that emerge, where change is made possible.

### Complementarity

Dyads, couples, and systems tend to get stuck in complementary relations. Complementarity is characterized by splitting in which one side takes a position complementary to—the opposite of—the other side. If one is experienced as "the doer," then the other becomes the "done to" (Benjamin, 2018, p. 24); if one is the victim, then the other becomes the victimizer; if one is active, then the other becomes passive; and so on. Polarities are split between the two members, and the more each one locks into a singular position, the more rigidly the other is locked into the opposing, complementary position, thus heightening the splitting and tightening the polarization.

### Enactment

A broad definition of enactment is an event within the therapeutic process where the patient and the therapist unconsciously become caught up in a deep emotional impasse involving dissociated affective states, occurring within both parties. These dissociated states are most often related to unworked issues of aggression or eroticism. In an enactment, the action of complementarity—doer and done to—dominates. When this happens, both parties within the dyad feel unrecognized and under the sway of the other's power, believing that the only response can be submission or resistance.

Enactment is considered by some theorists as discrete (Maroda, 2022), as continuous and ubiquitous (Bohleber et al., 2017), and as a part of the ordinary ebb and flow of analytic life (small "e") or as highly condensed unconscious psychic elements of heightened attention that take hold of analytic activity for periods of time (big "E") (Bass, 2003). Karen Maroda (2022) cautions the overuse of enactment and differentiates enactment as a "discrete, observable event that is affect-driven, characterized by a lack of awareness and frequently discombobulating" (p. 122). Maroda also directs us to Lew Aron's more nuanced view where he felt that to refer to enactment only as discrete is too limiting, while at the same time, he cautions us to not view enactment so broadly that all of analysis sinks into one big enactment (Maroda, p. 121).

So then, what is it? From my own point of view, when we reserve enactment only as a discrete event, we risk ignoring the fact that from the very first encounter, the unconscious-to-unconscious of the two subjects—therapist and patient—is immediately activated. From the beginning, the unconscious is evoked within our viscera, our minds, and our bodies. Indeed, there are discrete notable events that shock and mark the treatment in a particular way, experiencing a shift from the telling of story to being in the story. But what can be experienced as seismic shifts within the treatment have also been present all along, either being ignored or unconsciously readying itself for expression. Whether or not enactment is viewed as both discrete and continuous, distinctive to enactment is: (1) an attempt to communicate an aspect of the patient's story that cannot be verbalized, (2) a convergence of two affective states emerging within both the therapist and the patient, (3) general consideration as an unconscious to unconscious experience, though it ebbs and flows in and out of awareness, (4) a provocation of dissociated psychic content that both patient and therapist have avoided, and (5) a time where the therapist unconsciously acts in accordance to the disassociated parts of the patient's past.

For example, when a patient cannot access parts of themselves and has yet to acquire the capacity to mentalize and reflect upon the harm done, the patient unconsciously enacts the dissociated feelings with the therapist. When the therapist's own dissociated affective states are provoked in response to the patient's dissociated self-states, and the therapist lacks the capacity for reflection and disengages or blames the patient, the therapeutic dyad is caught in an enactment. These negative dissociated affective states are reflected in feelings such as disgust, guilt, fear, anxiety, and anger. These negative or unwanted emotions result in a collusion or collision. In colluding, enactments can go on interminably, as the patient and therapist continue to use the other to work out their own personal, dissociated self-states. Colluding occurs when the therapist is unable to reflect upon how their feelings, actions, and interactions relate to the patient's story and fails to invite the patient to do the same. When the therapeutic couple is able to reflect and give language and meaning to the enactment, the treatment is advanced (see discussion of the Third below). Perhaps a way to consider the discrete from the continuous is that the analytic pair in reliving the patient's story in direct relationship to the therapist, is in a continuous flow of repetition of their intrapsychic and interpersonal life. A discrete enactment would be when the patient and the therapist are resistant to and defending against these repetitions and eventually the resistance between the two explodes. This is perhaps why we talk about enactments as inevitable, powerful, and rich with potential for significant growth.

As therapists, we read others by attending to our bodies and what we are feeling in their presence and by attending to their facial expressions, body movements, inflections, and tone of voice. But it is an imperfect read. Though we might be quite good at reading the other, our reads need verifying. It is in the working through of our misreads where most psychotherapy takes place. Feiner (1988) states:

> In the end the patient uses the analyst's failures, often quite small ones, perhaps maneuvered by the patient and we have to put up with being misunderstood even hated…it is the failure…that is singled out as important on account of its being a reproduction of the original and [it is the failure and through the repair] that will create new growth.
>
> (p. 645)

It is essential to understand that enactments are not mistakes but strivings for a higher level of growth and organization, and their negotiations are a function of the developing and emerging relationship. The processing of each person's implicit self/selves within the relationship provides the raw material for new experiences, new actions, and new meanings for both parties. The intersubjective process of joining and co-creation cannot be defined, identified, or predicted ahead of time, because it occurs within the context of what transpires unexpectedly and thus requires a leap into the unknown. Enactments are considered a way of contact, a vital spark and embodiment (Ulanov, 2009). Enactment is understood to be that place where the patient's inner life becomes vividly animated, activating deep emotional reactions within the therapist. If the analytic couple can hold on and work it through, access to deeper reflection, insight, dialogue and negotiation (*the Third*) are made possible. If not, the therapy falters and either comes to an end or enters into a conjoint accommodation—where both therapist and patient avoid further affective arousals and conflicts.

### The Third

When two separate subjects interact, the thoughts, feelings, and bodily sensations co-created between the two become a subject within itself. Two separate subjectivities produce a third entity beyond their own individual subjectivities. This third entity/subject is akin to Buber's notion of the "in-between," contemporary psychoanalysis' use of "field theory," and Winnicott's conception of "potential space." This in-between space, generated by two subjects, is the space of psychic energy and of therapeutic process. The Third:

> is an effort to create a psychic space within which to think together about ways in which patient and analyst are similar and different, merged and separate, identified and differentiated…a place where they are able to achieve a *third* (italics mine) position, beyond a

transference-countertransference interlock [and] binary thinking into a transitional, symbolic space of thirdness and intersubjectivity.

(Aron, in Barsness, 2018, p. 122)

Though this Third space emerges from onset of two subjects meeting, creating, negating, persevering, and preserving (Ogden, 1986), Jessica Benjamin (2018) differs with Ogden understanding the Third as a space that is co-created between two subjectivities and must be achieved. For Benjamin, the Third is an effort to create a psychic space (in contrast to Ogden who states the psychic space exists in and of itself) within which to think together about ways in which the patient and analyst are similar and different. She refers to the Rhythmic Third as merged, in-sync, one-ness; the Differentiating Third refers to two-ness, or the capacity to hold the other in their uniqueness, the capacity to hold the tension of differentness. It is the ability to hold a position from more than one perspective. Benjamin (2018) states, "the third is a position constituted through holding the tension of recognition between difference and sameness, taking the other to be a separate but equivalent center of initiative and consciousness with whom nonetheless feelings and intentions can be shared" (p. 4). The Third space in Buber's philosophy is when the subject *turns* toward the other as a Thou and where genuine meeting is potentialized. For Carl Jung, it is when two opposing forces (two separate subjectivities) can co-exist that a third way will emerge.

*Forgiveness and the Third*

The act of forgiveness is complex, and the study of forgiveness within the field of psychology is new yet seems related to understanding the third and mutual recognition. Forgiveness has been perceived and spoken of within the realm of the religious and reluctantly integrated into psychoanalytic thought. However, as the growth of a person in psychoanalytic theory is predicated upon one's capacity to relinquish and reconcile the captivity of their past, the study of forgiveness is deemed essential to psychodynamic/analytic study. From our dialectical lens (the capacity to hold opposing views/experiences in tension), the use of the analytic Third (breaking out of the binary of doer and done to), and multiple self-theory (integration of multiple self-states, including one's own potential to harm), it perhaps could be said that the act of forgiveness lies at the very core of relational psychoanalytic/psychodynamic theory and practice.

In this complex task of forgiving, the psyche is liberated from the introjects of negative, ensnared self-states associated with the harm that has been inflicted. Forgiveness gradually shifts the patient's focus from the perpetrator [offender] to the trauma [wound] itself, a shift, poet David Whyte (2021) writes, from attacking and blaming the wrongdoer to a focus on the sadness and the plethora of other painful feelings associated with the circumstances… and the focus on the painfulness of those circumstances rather than on how could he/she have done this or that to me (p. 25). He goes on to say:

> To forgive is to assume a larger identity than the person who was first hurt, to mature and bring to fruition an identity that can put its arm, not only around the afflicted one within but also around the memories seared within us by the original blow and through a kind of psychological virtuosity, extend our understanding to one who first delivered it.
>
> (p. 43)

This shift is consistent with the emphasis in psychodynamic theory that prioritizes affective states over cognitive configurations. The operative phrase is "gradually shifts," because redeeming the hurt, the wound, the sting, the trauma, requires remembering. As we remember, we rage and ache. We ache because the harm that has been committed not only "refuses to eliminate the original wound but draws us closer to its source" (Whyte 2021, p. 23). The source is often someone we thought we could trust, who would love, rather than harm. The source can also be a violation, an injustice, a misunderstanding. The source, in whatever form, lives on in a person's mind and heart, developing into self-states of hurt, anger, vengeance, dissociation, depression, and anxiety. To forgive requires remembering. Remembering leads to reliving, reliving leads to grief, grief leads to mourning and to the question of whether one can forgive.

The most common practice in psychotherapy is assisting patients toward recognition and ultimately resolution of their past. The resolve results in the patient's capacity to relinquish negative affective states brought forth by violations/injustices that have harmed, as well as the unconscious wish of entitlement, such as "this should never have happened to me" (Benjamin, 2018, p. 25) and the wish for confession and reconciliation. This letting go, in and of itself, is a significant feat.

However, we are created in relationships, formed in relationship, harmed in relationship, and healed in relationship. Consequently, the reality of interconnectedness and the desire to be restored, often denied, to those with whom we have been harmed, lingers. Therefore, regardless of the lack of reciprocity from the wrongdoer, the desire for reconciliation is a universal, fundamental relational wish. Persons are relational beings, motivated by the desire to be healed and to be a healer—to understand and to value. Forgiveness, then, is not only a letting go of deeply held negative affective states but also a re-entering into the broken/wounded and/or traumatized relationship, either directly and/or within a therapeutic relationship. The act of forgiveness, in fact:

> involves the individual's unconscious wish and drive to reclaim his basic entitlement to specific, extremely significant relationships of which he has been deprived. It is not a rejection of anger, a suspension of judgment…a relinquishing of fear—fear of being re-traumatized—and of the defenses that accompany it. It is the willing re-establishment of a bond once shattered by failure driven by the wish for reinvestment in the psychic value of the offender.
>
> (Benjamin, 2018, p. 242)

Reinvestment offers the possibility of reconciliation through mutual recognition. However, investing in the psychic value of the offender does not always result in reconnection. Understanding the various levels of trauma inflicted and the psychological capacity of the person who has been harmed, it is recognized that reconciliation/mutual recognition may not be possible. In such cases, restoration is determined, whereby the identity of the one who has been harmed is no longer dictated by the one who has harmed.

As difficult as it may be, acknowledging the perpetrating other as subject and as co-human results in agency empowerment for the victim. What is meant by agency is that the person (the victim) transforms the betrayal by taking initiative. In taking charge of the offense, the power dynamic shifts. Agency exists when the betrayed believes that the ability to repair—in whatever form that may take—is within their power.

The work of forgiveness understands that at the root of trauma/brokenness lies deep shame and fear of the other. To be relieved of shame and fear requires not only remembering, mourning, and acceptance—although these alone are a big achievement—but also, as noted, involves a reinvestment in the broken relationship. In the process of reinvestment, there is a fear that in forgiving the offender, one must forget. However, forgiveness does not occlude harm done and forgetting; rather, it holds the harm in tension rather than falsely obliterating it through denial, dismissal, or vengeance. It remembers, while it also re-imagines. By breaking through the defensive actions of splitting and projection and confronting the polarity that it can be "only one or the other" or that "only one can live," an alternative action (the Third) is potentialized. In this third space, the binary of perpetrator/victim is disrupted and the capacity to hold the tension and complexity of both/and is advanced.

This third space breaks down binaries and potentiates what Buber (2003) refers to as "deep calling unto deep" (p. 46)—that is, to that part of our co-humanity that seeks relatedness over destructiveness. Forgiveness changes not only the heart of the forgiver but also their responsiveness toward the offender. Though relatedness/reconciliation may not always be achieved, through relating to the harm through remembering, mourning the loss of what shouldn't have been; relinquishing the ongoing desire of what could be; recognizing the offender's humanity and relating to the offender as subject rather than object; and recognizing one's own propensity to harm, the passive victim position is resituated, and relatedness revitalized.

Our job as therapists in facilitating a movement toward forgiveness recognizes that forgiveness is mostly an *action*, not an *act*, and takes place over time. We also recognize that the *action* of forgiveness is dependent upon a witness—that is, someone who acknowledges the harm that has been committed and joins with the patient in processing the attendant emotions that may replicate themselves in the therapeutic process. Through the therapeutic process, it is hoped that the stuckness created by the binaries of either/or perpetrator/victim are disrupted.

*Mutual Recognition*

Mutual recognition involves an affective meaningful experience of the other not as an object to control, resist, consume, or push away, but as another mind to work with: "An essential point of recognition theory is the awareness of the other as subject rather than object" (Benjamin, 2018, p. 10). Martin Buber refers to this as *turning* away from self-referencing, concerned with only one's "me-ness," toward the other as subject. An outcome of psychotherapy is where the "subject gradually becomes able to recognize the other person's subjectivity, developing the capacity for attunement and tolerance of difference" (p. 15). This is an interesting turn in the psychotherapy process where the two subjects, both patient and therapist, confirm the other. The therapist's willingness to be recognized by the patient is part of the healing.

## Theoretical Foundation Two: Interpersonal Neurobiology

Interpersonal neurobiology explores the effect that relationships have on the brain and how the quality of interpersonal interactions directly impacts affect regulation and the creation of new patterns of relating. The brain has multiple neuron systems that manifest as physical changes in neural structures of the brain and affect regulation. Schore (2018) states that "regulation theory dictates that in heightened affective moments, the patient's unconscious internal working model of attachment, whether secure or insecure, is reactivated in right-lateralized implicitly procedural memory and re-enacted in the psychotherapeutic relationship" (p. 245). Disruptions to the continuity, presence, and availability of the primary caregivers plays a central role in psychoneuropathogenesis. These primary relational configurations register in the brain, mirror neuron to mirror neuron, situated in the neocortex forming one's mind about the interaction. The idea of mirroring another's affective experience assists in assimilation and in differentiation as we begin to form a mind about our relationship to the other and to our environment.

These encounters are downloaded as representations and not necessarily truths but are experienced through the lens of wishes, fantasies, dreams, and desires formed because of earlier formative experiences. Relational configurations, including the self, the object, and the psychological space in-between, are referred to as intersubjective space. Thus, interpersonal relations are the building blocks of the mind, determining our attitudes, perceptions, reactions, and feelings. New experiences stimulate neural activity and interrupt old patterns of perceptions. Thus, the brain and the mind are seen as both stubborn and fluid, and the self or the mind is not seen as a structure outside the interpersonal field.

The left brain's function is that of explicit knowledge, language, and the capacity to organize thoughts and feelings. It is logical, calculating, analytical, and interested in outcomes and processes; it is the conscious self. The right brain is referred to as the seat of our emotions and is activated through our intuition, multiple affective states, and imagination. It is the felt sense of who we are as a person. The right brain is the first to develop as it precedes language and is mediated through nonverbal, intuitive relational contact and thus is unconscious. "Attachment trauma is imprinted in right cortical-sub-cortical systems, encoding disorganized-disoriented insecure internal working models that are non-consciously accessed at later points of interpersonal emotional distress" (Schore, 2018, p. 245). Affect regulation/dysregulation is mediated between right-brain to right-brain synchronous and asynchronous interactions.

Affective states between the right brains of the patient and therapist are best described as intersubjectivity. The right-brain processes are reciprocally activated on both sides of the therapeutic alliance. These unconscious non-verbal expressions are felt before they are thought. Right-brain processes are reciprocally activated on both sides and impact regulation and dysregulation of affect. Working through ruptures, interlocks, and enactments shifts the chemistry of the brain, "Emotions are deepened in intensity and sustained in time when they are intersubjectively shared [occurring] in moments of deep contact" (Schore, 2018, p. 246).

## Theoretical Foundation Three: Buber and the Philosophy of I/Thou

A quick read of Buber often leaves the reader thinking the I/Thou encounter is simply a moment of meeting when two people come to understand the other and relational tension is released. But the I/Thou moment is not encountered through sameness, agreement, or compromise; rather, it is predicated on the recognition of difference. A genuine encounter is the act of living in the ache and the beauty of contrast. It is the move from using the other as an object for personal gain and power. It is the act of *turning* toward the other as a (w)holy other. It is the hope that two separates can find unity in contrast.

- **I-Thou/I-It:** (*Thou*) is understood as a relationship. Rather than approaching the other as an object (*It*), approaching the other as a Thou is an invitation for relationship. "Thou" points to the quality of a relationship that risks vulnerability and surrender and hopes for genuine meeting where the other turns reciprocally. The term "It" describes the world of categories, objects, and things we use, including others to accomplish what we must. But it is only in the realm of Thou that transformation of the self is made possible.
- **Confirmation:** Buber makes a distinction between *affirmation* and *confirmation*. He held that affirmation is the beginning of a relationship, but that real healing through genuine meeting demands confirmation. Confirmation is the experience of being known for who you are and open to who you will become. Buber, by clarifying affirmation and confirmation, sees confirmation as the "move from accepting the other as a person like myself, to specifically confirming the other in their unique historic, cultural or ethnic personhood, to validating the other's present stance and third

direction of movement into the future" (Kramer, 2003, p. 197). Confirmation comes through direct encounter with another person, where contrast and difference are valued and where transformation is made possible. Confirmation stands up for the other for who they are instead of what we may want them to be.

- **Turning:** Turning refers to the risk of turning toward the other with your whole being. Turning embodies what Buber says is a double movement, requiring a letting go of semblance and entering relationship with your entire being. Turning involves being fully present to the other and involves *contrast, imagining the real,* and *vital reciprocity*. The word "turning" emerges from Buber's Hasidic Jewish tradition and points back to God's glory as dwelling in every living thing. Each human being's purpose is to "bring forth the godliness in all things and to bring about the actualization of God's presence in all actions" (Kramer, 2003, p. 132).
- **Contrast:** Contrast is asymmetry. It refers to mutual presence, not like-mindedness. Buber makes it clear that a genuine encounter is predicated on difference. Genuine meeting occurs when persons in their differentiated selves are able to surrender to the other.
- **Imagining the Real:** Buber talks about Imagining the Real, an idea that in an I-Thou stance, we offer our minds toward the other and to what they might be wishing, feeling, perceiving, and thinking. We do so not in a detached manner, but as a genuine inquiry of their being. The idea Buber is getting at here is the effort/capacity to feel beyond a general discomfort of the other to actually feel the pain of the other: "This making present increases until it is a paradox in the soul when I and the other are embraced by a common living situation" (Buber, 1970, p. 14).
- **Vital Reciprocity:** Buber refers to this as presence of spontaneity and mutual presence.

### Theoretical Foundation Four: The Sacred

Many relationally oriented practitioners may not include the sacred as part of the theory. I have included it here as the sacred is an orienting aspect to my own understanding of relational theory. Also, whether one is religious or not, the idea of soul has been an aspect of psychoanalytic theory since Freud's time (psyche/soul), and I believe it hints at the inexplicable transcendent presence common to all human experience. Jungian analyst James Hillman (2020) describes the soul as that "which makes meaning possible, [deepens] events into experiences, is communicated in love, and has a religious concern. Through their varied rituals both psychoanalysis and religion have a shared teleology. Both seek meaning, depth, and purpose which is the work of the soul" (p. 52).

We live in a culture possessed with knowing and fixing, often leading to power differentials, splits, divisions, and hatreds. The need to know and to be certain about what we think we know often harms the other. In the movie

*Freud's Last Session*, there is a line, correctly or incorrectly ascribed to Freud, that says, "moral certainty is the beast." Indeed, it is, and we must be careful in our work to remain radically open to that which we do not understand and to what we fear. My understanding of the sacred is that it acknowledges not knowing and involves a recognition of the transcendent—something that is beyond ourselves. Also, within the sacred and inherent in most religions are concepts such as humility, love of neighbor, confession, forgiveness, and reconciliation—concepts embedded within RPT.

Though Freud saw religion as an illusion, a form of neurosis, and God as a fantasy based on an infantile need for a dominant father figure, he explored some of the deepest mysteries of the soul. He had a deep sense of suffering and of trauma, leaving his very dear friend, Swiss Pastor Oscar Pfister, to say to him:

> And he who through the creation of psychoanalysis has provided the instrument which freed suffering souls from their chains and opened the gates of their prison, so that they could hasten into the sunny land of a life-giving faith, is not far from the kingdom of God…Will you be angry with me if I see you, who have intercepted such glorious rays of the eternal light and exhausted yourself in the struggle for truth and human love, as closer, figuratively, to the throne of God, despite your alleged lack of belief, than many churchmen, mumbling prayers and carrying out ceremonies, but whose heart has never burned with knowledge and good will?
>
> (Pfister, 1913, in Freud, S. & Pifster, O.,1963), p. 86)

Freud, in one of his letters to Pfister (2019), wrote, "we know that by different routes we aspire to the same objectives for poor humanity" (p. 113). Professor Meng, editor of the Pfister/Freud letters, said that at the roots of both Pfister and Freud lay the love of truth and indeed love itself. Freud knew well that at the core of Oskar's religious faith was love. Although Freud claimed to be an atheist, Pfister believed that Freud's words contradicted atheism and that Freud's own words were close to the throne of God.

Freud's atheism has kept lively discussion of spirituality out of analytic discussions. One has to look deep to find such discourse, but they exist. One example is that of psychoanalyst Wilfred Bion who constructed a complicated mathematical grid to define the human mind. And yet, at the end of Bion's life, he no longer felt convinced of his earlier mathematical equations, turning his attention to what he called "O," a designation he used to define the unknown Other, the transcendent other that cannot be known or grasped.

These religious ideas align with RPT and its understanding of intersubjectivity that holds to the notion that the road to the patient's intrapsychic and interpersonal world is not through an objective review of the patient's story. There is an appreciation of the unknown, of suffering, and of honoring the dignity of the other. As we lend ourselves to deep affective states that infect and disrupt, we surrender our certitude, rendering ourselves vulnerable to the other. Our responsibility, according to McWilliams (2004), is to remain "open, uncertain, unknowing, without memory or desire, and essentially unconscious enabling the patient to gain access to the analyst's own unconscious mental functioning in a way that generates emotional intimacy of a highly unusual kind" (p. 42). McWilliams' words can be summed up in the word *surrender*, where there is an absence of domination, control, and certainty. In the Christian tradition, this is exampled in the person of Christ, who "though being in the very nature of God, did not consider equality with God to be grasped and taking on the nature of a servant humbled himself and became obedient to death for the sake of all" (NSRV, Philippians, 2:6–8). Surrender gives up position, privilege, and prerogatives, relinquishing all for the sake of the other.

This stance of offering space for otherness, a space of humility and receptivity to the will and life of another, is a kenotic (self-emptying) act. The fundamental action of kenosis refers to the embrace of what is often the intolerable, establishing our real character when we dare to defend against the compulsion to defend or destroy. Even more, it dares to offer love as a possibility of growth. The key characteristic of the kenotic community is solidarity, not separation. In the Jewish Hasidic tradition, the biblical term *teshuvah* (turning to God), the word turning emerges from and points back to God's glory as dwelling in every living thing. Each human being's purpose is to bring about the actualization of God's presence in all actions.

This aligns with the theory of intersubjectivity and mutual recognition: "A position that believes positive outcome is the capacity to see others as equal subjects...and the reciprocating experience of the other's acknowledgement of oneself" (Hoffman, 1983, p. 386). This notion aligns with Buber's I/Thou, where "genuine meeting occurs when people enter dynamic solidarity with one another...and this deep bonding is contained neither in one, nor the other, nor in the sum of both, but becomes present between them... through directness and wholeness, will and grace, and the presence of mutuality" (Kramer, p. 20). Jürgen Moltmann (1993) refers to this meeting as the "intimate indwelling and complete interpenetration of the persons in one another...and that by their eternal love, the divine person exists so intimately with one another, for one another and in one another that they constitute themselves in their unique, incomparable and complete unity" (p. 156).

G. K. Chesterton (1925) wrote the following parable:

A man who was entirely careless of spiritual affairs died and went to hell. And he was much missed on earth by his old friends. His business agent went down to the gates of hell to see if there was any chance of bringing him back. But though he pleaded for the gates to be opened, the iron bars never yielded. His priest also went and argued: "He was not really a bad fellow; given time he would have matured. Let him out, please!" The gate remained stubbornly shut against all their voices. Finally, his mother came; she did not beg for his release. Quietly, and with a strange catch in her voice, she said to Satan: "Let me in." Immediately the great doors swung open upon their hinges. For love goes down through the gates of hell and there redeems the dead.

(p. 149)

It seems that in our work there is a willingness to go down into the depths of hell of our patients and tarry with, rather than observe from beyond, and to become most well at our points of surrender—in those deconstructed moments when we fall upon our knees and cry "holy," not in an illusory haze but in wonder, in awe, and in hope of the mystery of our very being.

At the core of psychodynamic therapy and religion is "let me in."

And when we go this far, we are often left on the edge of something we cannot fathom or know, and we find relief in the beauty of not knowing, of letting go, and being open to the sacred surprises of the Universe.

## References

Aron, L. (2018) Core Competency Four: Relational Dynamic: The There and Then and the Here and Now. In R.E. Barsness, (Ed), *Core Competencies in Relational Psychoanalysis: A guide to practice, study and research*. London. Routledge

Atwood, G., Brandchaft, B., & Stolorow, R. (1987). *Psychoanalytic treatment: An intersubjective approach*. Hillsdale, NJ: The Analytic Press.

Barsness, R. E. (2018). *Core competencies of relational psychoanalysis: A guide to practice, study and research*. London: Routledge.

Barsness, R. E., & Strawn, B. (2018). Courageous speech/disciplined spontaneity. In R. E. Barsness (Ed.), *Core competencies in relational psychoanalysis: A guide to practice, study and research* (Chapter 10, pp. 179–200). London: Routledge.

Bass, A. (2003). "E" enactments in psychoanalysis another medium, another message. *Psychoanalytic Dialogues, 13*(5), 657–675.

Benjamin, J. (2018). *Beyond doer and done to: Recognition theory, intersubjectivity and the Third*. London: Routledge.

Bible New Revised Standard Version. (1990). Zondervan.

Bohleber, W., Fonagy, P., Jimenez, J. P., Scarfone, D., Varvin, S., & Zysman, S. (2017). Towards a better use of psychoanalytic concepts: A model illustrated using the concept of enactment. *International Journal of Psychoanalysis, 94*(3), 501–530.

Bollas, C. (2017). *The shadow of the object: Psychoanalysis of the unthought known*. New York: Columbia Press.

Bromberg, P. (1993). Shadow and substance: A relational perspective on clinical process. *Psychoanalytic Psychology, 10*(2), 166.

Buber, M. (2003). *I and thou* (R. G. Smith, Trans.). Continuum. (Original work published 1923)

Chesterton, G. K. (1925). *The everlasting man*. London: Hodder & Stoughton.

Cornelius, J. T. (2018). The case for psychoanalysis: Exploring the scientific evidence. In R. E. Barsness (Ed.), *Core competencies in relational psychoanalysis: A guide to practice, study and research* (Chapter 2, pp. 24–43). London: Routledge.

Feiner, A. (1988). Countertransference and misreading – The influence of the anxiety of misreading. *Contemporary Psychoanalysis, 24*, 612–650.

Fosshage, J. (2000). The meaning of touch in psychoanalysis: A time for reassessment. *Psychoanalytic Inquiry, 20*, 21–43.

Freud, S., & Pfister, O. (1963). *Psychoanalysis and faith: The letters of Sigmund Freud and Oskar Pfister* (E. L. Freud & H. Meng, Eds.). Basic Books.

Gabbard, G. (1996). The analyst's contribution to the Erotic Transference. *Contemporary Psychoanalysis, 32*, 249–273.

Geist, R. (2009). Empathy, connectedness, and the evolution of boundaries in self psychological treatment. *International Journal of Psychoanalytic Self-Psychology, 4*, 165–180.

Grossmark, R. (2018). *The unobtrusive analyst*. London: Routledge.

Hillman, J. (2020). *The soul's code*. Portland, OR: Blackstone Press.

Hoffman, I. Z. (1983). The patient as interpreter of the analyst's experience. *Contemporary Psychoanalysis, 19*, 389–423.

Kramer, P. (2003). *Martin Buber's I and Thou: Practicing living dialogue*. Mahwah, NJ: Paulist Press.

Kuchuck, S. (2021). *The relational revolution*. London: Confer.

Maroda, K. J. (2004). *The power of countertransference: Innovations in analytic technique*. London. Routledge.

Maroda, K. (2018). *The power of countertransference: Innovations in analytic technique*. London: Routledge.

Maroda, K. (2022). *The analyst's vulnerability: Impact on theory and practice*. Routledge.

McWilliams, N. (2004). *Psychoanalytic psychotherapy: A practitioners guide*. New York: Guildford Press.

McWilliams, N. (2016). Psychoanalysis. In I. Marini & M. A. Stebnicki (Eds.), *The professional counselor's desk reference* (2nd ed., pp. 183–189). N.Y. Springer Publishing Company.

Meng, H., & Freud, E. L. (1963). *Psychoanalysis and faith: The letters of Sigmund Freud and Oskar Pfister*. New York: Basic Books.

Mitchell, S. A. (1984). Object relations theories and the developmental tilt. *Contemporary Psychoanalysis, 20*(4), 473–499.

Mitchell, S. (1988). *Relational concepts in psychoanalysis*. Cambridge, MA: Harvard University Press.

Mitchell, S. A. (1993). *Hope and dread in psychoanalysis*. New York: Basic Books.

Moltmann, J. (1993). *Trinity and the Kingdom*. Minneapolis, MN: Fortress Press.

Morrison, T. (1997). *Song of Solomon*. New York: Vintage.

Norcross, J. C., & Lambert, M. (2018). Psychotherapy relationships that work III. *Psychotherapy, 55*(4), 303–315.

Ogden, T. H. (1986). *The matrix of the mind*. Northvale, NJ: Aronson.

Orange, D. M. (1995). *Emotional understanding: Studies in psychoanalytic epistemology*. New York: Guilford Press.

Rolheiser, R. (2010). Touching our loved ones inside the body of Christ. *St. Anthony Messenger, 118*(9), 44–45. https://example.com

Schore, A. (2018). The right brain and psychoanalysis. In R. E. Barsness (Ed.), *Core competencies in relational psychoanalysis: A guide to practice, study and research* (Chapter 13, pp. 241–282). London: Routledge.

Ulanov, A. (2009). Countertransference and the erotic. *Journal of Religion and Health, 48*, 90–96.

Whyte, D. (2012). *Consolations*. Langley, WA: Many Rivers Press.

Winnicott, D. W. (1971). *Playing and reality*. Routledge.

Winnicott, D. W. (1986). *Home is where we start from*. New York: Norton.

# 3 Core Competencies (Disciplines) in Relational Psychoanalysis

## A Summary

In this chapter, I offer a clinical framework useful for conducting relational psychodynamic treatment and applicable within the relational psychodynamic supervision model presented in this book. This chapter summarizes a qualitative research study I conducted that identified seven core competencies representative of relational psychoanalysis. While it is nearly impossible to encapsulate the full breadth of theory and practice within psychoanalysis—a bold aim of the study—these competencies provide a common scaffolding to guide us in our uniqueness. The research culminated in the publication of the edited text: *Core Competencies in Relational Psychoanalysis: A Guide to Practice, Study and Research* (2018). In this chapter, I will summarize each of these seven competencies: therapeutic intent; therapeutic stance/attitude; deep listening and affective attunement; the relational dynamic—the there and then and the here and now; patterning and linking; repetition and working through; and courageous speech/disciplined spontaneity and will discuss the overarching category of these competencies which is love. In the text of this chapter, I have recast the word competencies to the word disciplines as the term discipline better aligns with what we do as relational therapists. Guided by theory and experience, we continually discipline ourselves to enhance our knowledge and clinical skills. It is a life-long work. Competency, on the other hand, suggests a sense of arrival and completion.

It is hoped that this structure, when used as a regular discipline of practice, will guide and sustain the clinician in their work and are the disciplines underlying the MAMAL method of supervision.

## Core Discipline One: Therapeutic Intent

Steve Tublin (2018) states,

> rendering one's intent explicit compels the analyst to know, as much as that is possible, what they consider essential to a satisfying existence, what sort of mind they believe allows for the creation of such a life and what they are capable of doing, via the ritualized application of their craft to advance that aim.
>
> (p. 83)

DOI: 10.4324/9781003532828-3

Psychoanalytic practice is thus first and foremost informed by therapeutic intent. Emmanuel Ghent in his seminal paper, Credo, states, "ultimately a belief system that the analyst lives and works by…makes a very significant difference as to how one hears, what one hears, how one assembles what is heard, and how one conducts oneself in the analytic setting" (Ghent, 1989, p. 170). Analytic clinicians orient their work toward outcomes informed by what we believe constitutes change. Having a coherent understanding of the goal of treatment, therapeutic action is better able to be determined. Comedian Michael Jr. (2016) challenges us saying, "when you know your why you have options on what your what can be" (Michael Jr: Know Your Why—YouTube).

In contrast to behavioral models, which provide clear therapeutic outcomes and manualized treatments to meet those outcomes, working analytically is far more fluid and much more difficult to express. Cognitive-behavioral techniques, more clearly spell out what one can expect from a particular treatment, such as symptom management, reduction in cognitive distortions, and anger management. However, when psychodynamic therapists are asked about the outcomes of a psychodynamic treatment, they often feel stumped for an answer. However, their answer is important not only for the patient to know what to expect in treatment but also as important for the therapist to know to guide them in their work.

In contrast to an emphasis on behavior, core to a psychoanalytic outcome is development of the self of the person and particularly, how they navigate relationally in their world. A desired outcome of a psychoanalytic treatment is the vitalization of the human person. Our manual is the therapeutic relationship.

Winnicott surmised that a person can be normal without being alive. Second-century mystic St. Irenaeus says, "the Glory of God is persons fully alive!" Most of us don't live fully alive. Many people live with a sort of low-level depression, lack vitality, and are detached from or deny important aspects of their emotional life. While persons may seek treatment to resolve a particular behavioral issue, the underlying issue of their pain is generally a lack of connectedness to their emotional and relational life. Nancy McWilliams in her book, *Psychoanalytic Supervision* (2021), speaks of this lack of vitality as "living in a state of 'as-if-ness' and further quotes Helene Deutschs (1944) concept of the non-vital self "'as-if personality,' Winnicott's (1960) "false self," Joyce McDougalls (1980) term the 'normopath, and Christopher Bollas (1987) [viewed these prolonged states of dissociation from a person's affective life] as the 'normotic" (p. 63).

Our work seeks to interrupt this apathy. Thus, our why as to why we do this work is to assist our patients to live a full and meaningful life. To move beyond a life of "as-if-ness." To assist them to live and think creatively, openly and with imagination. To increase their ability to live with uncertainty, engage robustly, with risk, knowing they will be hurt, feel shame, make errors, collapse at times but possess the will to live on. To fully enter into the complications, the pain, the agony and the ecstasy of human relations, with love and hate, and an attitude of redemption and restoration.

Following the publication of the text and my use of it in the classroom, I was delighted when a student in their first internship, enthusiastically emailed me telling me how having at hand the disciplines assisted her in keeping a patient she wished to work with, that her supervisor had denied her, because she did not have CBT training. The intern concurred with her supervisor that she wasn't trained in CBT but wished to demonstrate her psychodynamic training and how she would approach her work with the patient. She began her conversation by outlining what she believed the outcome (therapeutic intent) of a psychodynamic treatment would provide and then detailed how various disciplines a stance of openness and curiosity; deep listening/affective attunement; working replications; the patterns that would emerge, linking them to the patient's past and present; attend to the potential conflicts that might arise and would do her best to be honest and sincere with her patient. The supervisor was impressed and proceeded to assign her the case. The intern knew her "why!" And because she knew her why, she figured out her how. When we know our why, we can, just as the intern was able to do, explain our how.

One of the primary concerns in psychoanalytic work is the lack of clarity about our treatment outcomes. Historically, we have assumed that insight into one's past, achieved through the analysis of the unconscious, interpretation of transference, and defensive structures, would lead to relief. However, in the relational psychodynamic trend and related research, we see that insight alone is insufficient. Instead, the vitalization of the self in direct relationship with the therapist is what creates significant shifts in the self. Vitalization replaces insight alone.

A student once asked me, "but isn't the therapeutic outcome to be guided by what the patient is seeking?" Yes, but only in part. We, the therapist, must first know what we believe and what we can provide and what we cannot provide. Knowing *our* why directs and informs us how we behave and work within an analytic setting. Knowing our why also guides us back to our purpose when we become confused or lost in the treatment process and helps us evaluate our progress over time.

A new patient once said, "I am here because I want my anxiety to go away, either by medication or by some psychological tips to stop the feeling." I responded that I do not provide medication and only infrequently give tips. I continued that since his life in general seemed to be functioning fairly well (meaning no immediate crisis), I was most interested in following his anxiety to its root, rather than just getting rid of it. I explained that our conversations would explore how his anxiety was exhibiting and inhibiting itself in his life and in his direct relationship with me. He decided to continue the treatment.

As we progressed, we discovered his anxious attachment to his mother and his anger toward a demanding father who expected perfection, and continued to be a strong influence in his life. We also noted his resistance to attaching to me and the therapeutic process, which was expressed in a "go away, come closer" interplay between us. By working through the evolving therapeutic relationship and the patient's historical formations, his dissociation from his affective states began to give way. He started facing and working through emotional losses, experiencing a more expansive range of emotions, including anxiety, but with an increased capacity to engage with and learn from them.

I share this case to illustrate that my understanding of a positive therapeutic outcome (i.e., vitalization, the capacity to experience multiple affective states, enjoyment of the full range of emotion, a more creative imagination of one's emotional life, and linking one's past formations with present patterns) guided my process. This understanding prevented me from being swayed into merely providing symptom reduction, which, though helpful in the short term, would not have addressed the long-term goal of vitalization. Knowing my why directed me in providing the treatment that I am able to offer and what I have expertise in. It is crucial for therapists to know their own expected outcomes and to clearly inform patients about these outcomes and the process to achieve them. It is in the interplay of what the patient wants and what the therapist can give which forms and informs the therapeutic process.

Knowing your why…shapes your how.

## Core Discipline Two: Therapeutic Stance/Attitude

Stephen Mitchell (2000) states, "The relational analyst's stance is quite different than earlier generations…the standard is not objectivity or rationality, but candor, openness and authenticity. The goal is not to circumvent influence, but continually to deconstruct or reflect upon int. The analyst's contribution is important not for its transcendent correctness, but for the genuineness of its self-reflective reports on the interaction with the patient" (p. 139).

Relational psychoanalysis was born out of radical critique of the authoritarian stance. From a relational perspective the therapist's stance is understood to be co-constructed where authority resides in the understanding and working through of what transpires in the relational dynamics that emerge between the therapist and the patients' interactions. Nancy McWilliams (2018) claims therapists should understand that we hold "authority about process but uncertainty about content" (p. 87). The process requires a stance of curiosity and awe, the use of the therapists' affective states elicited within the therapist in relation to the patient, a deep listening, emotional risk-taking, working with repetition, conflict and authenticity.

Working within a relational psychodynamic model, the self of the therapist is far more exposed than the psychoanalyst of the past. No longer protected by the luxury of anonymity, we are left with a greater responsibility of becoming radically open to our own subjectivity within the therapeutic dyad. Though we are taught to be radically open to our patient's narratives, we find our patients within ourselves requiring that we must undergo a "critical personal experience [in order] to deeply comprehend the patient's psychic reality" (Winnicott, 1949, p. 243). We must have an awareness and acceptance of our own human condition, our strengths, our flaws, our fears, our shame, and frankly, a humility that connects with the challenge of simply being human to understand our patients. Being capable of being open to our patients is directly related to how open we are toward ourselves. To work from a relational psychodynamic perspective, one's own subjectivity is activated and is actively involved throughout the therapeutic process.

In Chapter 4 of this text entitled: *The Essential I*, we will further explore the concept of radical openness of the therapist's self and the critical importance of the use of the therapist's self in the psychodynamic treatment.

## Core Discipline Three: Deep Listening/Affective Attunement

Deep Listening is an art form created over time. Because to fully attune to another's story "requires deep immersion within the transference-countertransference, an intersubjective experience that can only be made use of if the analyst can tolerate the uncertainty of a gradually unfolding narrative and can learn along the way the analyst's private nuanced, and embodied language that articulates the experience…The intimacy and intensity involved in this sort of psychoanalytic listening requires that we listen not only closely to our patients, but also… to ourselves-with-our-patients in the course of living within the emotional force field of dyadic analytic experience" (Griffen, 2016, p. 4).

Therapeutic listening is the sine qua non of most therapeutic approaches. What distinguishes the listening skills of the relational analyst, however, is what Reik called listening with the third ear, Singer called listening with one's viscera and Ogden reverie. My own understanding of listening is listening to the "conversation that is at hand," that is to the words that cannot found voice, and are experienced affectively, deep within our bodies, through unconscious messaging and in the patterns of relating that emerge within the therapeutic relationship.

The relational analyst listens for what the patient can no longer hear, deafened by their intellectual defenses that have built up walls around their emotional experiences. Therefore, the relational analyst seeks to be highly attuned, self-reflective and unguarded from their own defensive structures to free themselves to what is being stirred within them, knowing that through their own affective experience, they gain access to the patient's internal and external world, yet unknown or unspoken. Stuart Pizer (2018) says, "feeling tugged by the tension of tenderness in our deep affective involvement with what we recognize in the Other, both devoted and conflicted, we are moved to offer what we can of ourselves as therapists and analysts. As I have been defining the analyst's generous involvement it is not only an empathic witnessing, a 'being with.' [no], it entails a 'going forth' from within ourselves *toward* the patient's need" (p. 119).

Attending to affect, one is better able to enter the unconscious and disassociated aspects of the patient. The relational analyst prioritizes affect, recognizing that resonance at the emotional level is what leads to change.

## Core Discipline Four: The There and Then and the Here and Now

"History is not just fact and events. History is also a pain in the heart, and we repeat history until we are able to make another's pain in the heart our own" (Lester, 2005, Day of Tears—goodreads.com), and Eduardo Galeano (1992) says, "no history is mute. No matter how much they own it, break it, and lie about it, human history refuses to shut its mouth. Despite deafness and ignorance, the time that was continues to tick inside the time that is" (p. 25).

These two wise persons remind us that the history of *one* must penetrate the life of *another* in order for transformation to occur. History must not only be told, but also it must be lived. Freud's earliest contribution in recognizing human compulsion to repeat difficult and distressing experiences of earlier life continues to be not only true of all of us but also is central to an analytic treatment. Repetition appears in the relational landscape in the form of dreams, transferences, projections, enactments, denials. These therapeutic transactions are less about the pathologies of our patients (or of us) and are better understood as the only means the patient has at their disposal (at the moment) to make contact with another. Repetition is reaching out to the heart of another to be seen.

When repetition does not "hit" someone repetition has to continue until it does. Impasses within psychotherapy is often related to the therapist's unwillingness to participate in the repetition. It is only when the repetition activates affective states in the therapist and the therapist stays in the game and works it through with the patient that change is made possible. As Lester reminds, "we repeat history until we are able to make another's pain in the heart our own." If one cannot reach the other any change will be only on the surface. When the heart of the other is reached, it is then we can then talk of transformation.

Psychoanalysis has always recognized that past events, especially early developmental experiences, repeat themselves in the present. Therefore, relational analysts continue to attend to early attachment, developmental history, defensive structures, projections, transference and countertransference, asking themselves: "How has this person been shaped?" "What happened?" "What have they done with what happened?" Relational analysts, however, have expanded the emphasis on early parent-child relations, in particular the mother, to include other significant interpersonal relations as well as the influence of one's own culture and traumas that have shaped and formed a person's view of self.

Perhaps an even greater shift in relational theory is the attention to the "here and now" co-created between the patient and the analyst. In attending to this progression in analytic theory, analysts now consider such questions as: "What is being stirred in me?" "Why am I reacting in this way?" "How am I impacting this patient?" "Am I allowing myself to be fully immersed, with all my thoughts, all my feelings?" "What am I contributing within this relational milieu?" From this perspective, the relational analyst has modified the rationalistic interpretations of the Freudian era "from enlightening the patient about his life to helping him capture the nature of his emotional life in intimate detail [in direct relationship to the therapist having] moved from understanding and explaining of connections to concern with the present and an interest in immediate awareness of emotions" (Singer, 1970, p. 195).

The analyst's current view working in the here and now not only offers insight of the there and then but also an opportunity for a new relational experience. Thus, the analyst engages the patient in direct relationship with themselves, believing effective change comes from working through that which is co-created within the analytic dyad.

Historically, we have referred to the relational dynamic there-and-then-and-the-here-and-now as transference and countertransference. Relational psychodynamic theory moves beyond the binaries of transference/countertransference defining therapeutic space as way,

> to think together about ways in which patient and analyst are similar and different, merged and separate, identified and differentiated... a place where they are able to achieve a third position, beyond a transference-countertransference interlock [and] beyond binary thinking into transitional, symbolic space of thirdness and intersubjectivity.
>
> (Aron, 2018, p. 137)

Working within the intersubjective field shifts the emphasis of the treatment away from transference interpretation as the primary psychoanalytic technique to working directly within the therapeutic relationship addressing the inevitable impasses, enactments, inherent in a co-constructed intersubjective therapeutic relationship.

## Core Discipline Five: Patterning and Linking

Jazz musician, Ornette Coleman (1997), the innovative jazz musician, eloquently captured the complexity and multiplicity nature of the interpersonal rhythmic experience. He once remarked, "I'm having this conversation with you now. I'm talking, but I'm thinking, feeling, smelling, and moving. Yet I'm concentrating on what you're saying. So that means there's more things going on in the body than just the present thing that the person's got you doing." His words resonate with the idea that creativity emerges from a "rich tapestry of thoughts, emotions, and sensations" (p. 86).

The analyst not only considers recurring themes and patterns and how they may be linked to the past and repeated in the here and the now, as described in Discipline Four, the therapist attunes to the patterns that emerge within the analytic relationship itself. Psychoanalyst Steven Knoblauch speaks of concentrating on patterns of synchronicity and asynchronicity, trying to get a "sense" of the shifts and patterns that happen between the analyst and the patient concurrently wondering what these shifts might mean.

The linking of patterns within the analytic pair are often felt before they are known, appearing in the area of our brain (the right hemisphere) that registers at the feeling level. The research participants described patterning and linking by comments such as "I attend to the artistry of how I am with the patient in the moment." "Everything within the hour has some organizing principle." "The patterning is organic and artistic." "Both [patient and therapist] occupy roles; the question is how is it being played out?" "What is the relationship doing, what can I be doing with my patient, and what is the patient doing to me?" "What are the patterns that we are establishing?" "How are these patterns impacting us right now?" "What are the shifts that emerge through tone of voice, eye contact, bodily movements?"

Steven Knoblauch (2018), psychoanalyst and jazz musician, refers to patterning and linking as a "polyrhythmic weave," likening psychoanalysis to the music of the samba, "highlighting in the subtle micromoments of a clinical interaction… the emergent affective meanings that are being constituted within the rhythmic dialogue" (p. 143).

## Core Discipline Six: Repetition and Working Through

The role of conflict has always been a central theme in psychoanalysis. The relational perspective expands traditional psychoanalytic theories understanding of conflict however, holding to the view that understanding intrapsychic conflict in and of itself is insufficient. Believing deep change occurs at the emotional level, the relational analyst attends not only to intrapsychic conflict but also to the inevitable conflicts and impasses that emerge within the therapeutic relationship. Intrapsychic conflict has historically been revealed through interpretation and insight to one's past has served as the cure. In relational psychodynamic work, conflict is more front, and center as intrapsychic conflict is revealed interpersonally between the therapist and the patient and made available for analysis. Relational psychoanalytic treatment assumes interpersonal conflict and the working through of these differences, ruptures, entanglements, and enactments is central to the therapeutic process. "Although such ruptures of the alliance are the most stressful moments of the treatment, these "collisions of the therapist's and the patient's subjectivities also represent an intersubjective context of potential collaboration between their subjectivities, and thereby a context of interactive repair-a fundamental mental mechanism of therapeutic change" (Schore, 2018, p. 252).

Karen Maroda (1998) speaks to the inevitability of enactment—a co-constructed event involving both patient and therapist's past's—and its therapeutic potential. She says it is not only the patients past that is repeated but also "equally inevitable is the evocation of the analyst's past in terms of re-creating an emotional scenario [between the patient and the therapist]." She continues, "enactment is essentially an affective event. The action carries the purpose of fully expressing the intense emotion at the heart of the transference-countertransference exchange (p. 534). Though enactments have generally been thought of as an unconscious event, Maroda extends our understanding of enactment occurring not only unconsciously but also at the conscious level. She contends that strong emotional experiences within both therapist and patients, especially negative ones, are rarely out of awareness and though therapists tend to be conflict-avoidant, therapeutic change occurs by facing and facilitating the inevitable conflicts within the therapeutic relationship that arise.

As deep change occurs at the emotional level, presented relationally between the therapist and the patient, it is essential that the therapist attend to the conflicts that emerge in the relational dyad, holding to the view of the necessity of destruction, survival and recognition. At "the very foundation of psychoanalysis is that unconscious feelings and thoughts can be brought into awareness and expressed, [thus] creating the necessary conditions for working through" (Maroda, 2018, p. 170). It is in the working through, where the hope that one can survive is strengthened. "There can be no transforming of darkness into light and of apathy into movement without emotion" (Jung, 1969, http://jungcurrents.com).

### Core Discipline Seven: Courageous Speech/Disciplined Spontaneity

The relational analyst holds to the notion that a patient needs to hear what is on the therapist's mind and how the therapist experiences the patient. Therapists take risks by stating what has come to their mind within the context of the therapeutic relationship. Risky though their speech may be analysts offer their ideas from a non-authoritarian stance with curiosity and humility. Words are offered to the patient with a spirit of inquiry, exploration, and negotiation. Analysts consider their thoughts and affects and attempt to metabolize before they speak and while they are speaking. They are also willing to make a mistake in speaking, given their predisposition to follow the patient's response as the means for discovering understanding and meaning, rather than mere analytic interpretation. Interventions, thoughts, words come as conversations.

In the research study that formed my *Core Competencies* text (2018), participants spoke of courageous speech and disciplined spontaneity by stating that they do not operate from a script or from a formula. In fact, if they feel as though they are, they believe they may be missing or avoiding something. They live with the assumption that the encounter is unpredictable and unformulated and because of that, they must follow the experience of their patient in direct relationship to the experience of themselves. Phrases they used to describe analytic speech were, "Sometimes things just fly out of my mouth, which as long as I am there to explore this with the patient and it is connected to our experience, it is what is needed." "How do we know anything? By talking about what has happened." "I know that I can't have clarity unless I say something." "I recognize that because I am working with experience, the timing is always right because I am stating what it is that is happening." "I think that in some form the patient already knows what I am thinking anyway." "I do a lot of reflecting out loud. I suppose I am modeling the idea of looking inside while speaking outside."

When to speak and what to say remains challenging, but it is evident that the relational analyst chooses to let the patient in on their thoughts believing that in doing so, the work is advanced.

I was also struck by the risks these relational analysts were taking as well as the humility in which they offered their words. They said things such as, "psychoanalysis is a discipline of restraining oneself by being courageous enough to speak to what is happening." "Showing your emotions without being self-referential and maintaining the focus on the patient," and "speaking with curiosity, inquiry and exploration." It is about "wondering why I might wish to say something and why I may wish to not say something, I need to always consider my motivations." The analysts stated that there is a caution to be "mindful of the compulsion to interpret when I want to feel clever," and to "see this work as a mutual endeavor," and always to "remain open to surprise."

To speak courageously, the analyst must have a healthy respect for anxiety and tension without feeling threatened, hold direct requests for acknowledgement non-defensively and with curiosity, value their words as a means for exploration rather than as correctness, and finally follow how the therapeutic couple navigate what has been said...essentially, we play, we wonder and we ask, "has collaborative inquiry increased and is our patient freer to engage more deeply with themselves and with others?" (Barsness & Strawn, 2018, p. 198) and we remember, "to keep nothing back is the exact opposite of unreserved speech, [true authentic dialogue] is fulfilled in its being, between partners who have turned to one another in truth, who express themselves without reserve and are free of the desire for semblance, there is brought into being a memorable common fruitfulness which is found nowhere else" (Buber, 1947 as cited in Kaufmann, 1970 , p. 70).

## Core Discipline: Love

Though not all agree, I believe what lies at the heart of a psychoanalytic treatment is love. Though some analysts and therapists may balk at such an idea, I learned through my own research that to be faithful to the data that emerged from the analysts I interviewed that love was indeed the overarching category of the seven disciplines listed above. How so?

First, the majority of the interviewees stated unequivocally, "I love my patients."

Second, I found myself deeply moved by their expressions of joy, care, and compassion for their patients. I found myself touched by the intimacy of the cases that they shared, risking themselves emotionally and intellectually and wholeheartedly engaging the analytic process.

Third, as I was analyzing the data I began to see that the therapeutic relationship is a relationship founded upon a loving care act. A relationship that requires of themselves honesty and risk-taking, a deep immersion in the affective lives of the other, and devotion to scrutinize non-defensively their own selves in an attempt to understand, feel, and grasp the internal and interpersonal world of another. I found that the participants were willing to resist the urge for self-protection, surrender certainty, and engage in the inevitable conflicts, misrecognitions, and ruptures, and to stay in the conflict until the conflict is worked through. The analysts applied to themselves Freud's basic ethic of honesty, not only as an expectation that Freud believed an essential requirement for the patient. It is this honesty that births an unusual authenticity rarely found in human relations, and the primary factor that engenders change and transformation in our patients' lives. Daniel Shaw speaks of analytic love as a

> surrender to the process of building a therapeutic relationship…surrender of the need to know, of the need to be right, of the need to use our knowledge of the psyche and our position of authority to protect ourselves from being the one who needs help, by being instead the one who dispenses help. Analytic love encourages us to take risks with our patients, hoping that we are making productive choices but knowing that we may wound in the process. Analytic love is what protects us both…from the unfreedom of domination and submission. It is what supports both…in a sustained commitment to the intersubjective construction of the analytic relationship. Finally, analytic love contains the hope and the faith that where fear of retraumatization and alienation were, compassion, understanding, and mutuality shall be.
> (Shaw, 2014, pp. 148–149)

As I vetted my research and my wonderings about analytic love with other colleagues, I discovered that some analysts were uncomfortable with the word "love" and some even stated that they didn't love all of their patients, giving me pause to reconsider whether I was seeing love from a rose-colored lens and was it truly the overarching discipline of other seven disciplines? So how did it get included?

First, it was in the data—many reported their love for their patients and as I analyzed what analysts do, it was unavoidable that love was in the air. Second, as students in my Clinical courses were aware of the research I was conducting, and they knew that idea of love among analysts was controversial and of the conundrum of whether or not I would include analytic love as the core category.

In this two-semester class, there was a student who had said nothing during the entire course. Though he seemed engaged, I was curious about his silence. Now, at the end of the semester, having said our goodbyes, he approached me and quite intensely said: "Don't ever shy away from love…

you have brought it, you have lived it, I have bought it, and I believe it... and now, as a new practitioner, I have seen it. Don't ever give up on love." It shook me...and I believe he was the messenger I needed that sealed the deal on love as the essence of our work. It should be made clear that we don't decide to love a patient, and in fact, we know that alongside love negative affective states are not far behind and perhaps it is these multiple affective states that land us in the love we experience.

Daniel Shaw (2023) reflecting on Salvador Ferenczi's considerations on love says, that through his mutual analysis with Elizabeth Severn,

> analytic love was not something given by the analyst to the patient, but rather, that analytic love is co-constructed by the analytic couple when their work goes deep; when it has been honest enough to evoke mutual hate and survive it; and when in the process of repair, analyst and patient go on to become real to each other and therefore able to build mutuality – the kind of mutuality that Lewis Aron and Jessica Benjamin have described and termed intersubjective relatedness – relatedness that moves from binary subject-to-object relating into the co-created thirdness of subject-to-subject relating.
>
> (unpublished paper)

Love, truly, does not exploit. And the love of our patients is a love born out of a deep respect for the individual who comes to us in pursuit of recovering a shattered life because of trauma and harm. How can one not love and fully participate in such a pursuit?

## References

Aron, L. (2018). Chapter Seven: The there and then and the here and now. In R. Barsness (Ed.), *Core competencies in relational psychoanalysis a guide to practice, study, and research* (pp. 121–141). London: Routledge.

Barsness, R. (2018). *Core competencies in relational psychoanalysis a guide to practice, study, and research*. London: Routledge.

Barsness, R., & Strawn, B. (2018). Chapter Ten: Courageous speech/disciplined spontaneity. In R. Barsness (Ed.), *Core competencies in relational psychoanalysis a guide to practice, study, and research* (pp. 180–198). London: Routledge.

Bollas, C. (1987). *The shadow of the object: Psychoanalysis of the unthought known*. NY. Columbia University Press.

Buber, M. (1970). *I and thou* (W. Kaufmann, Trans.). Scribner.

Coleman, O. (1997). Interview by Jacques Derrida. In A. Norris (Ed.), *The new school: Conversations with the Avant-Garde* (p. 86). Chicago, IL: University of Chicago Press.

Deutsch, H. (1944). *The psychology of women: A psychoanalytic interpretation* (Vol. 1). NY. Green and Stratton.

Galeano, E. (1992). *Book of embraces*. New York: Norton.

Ghent, E. (1989). Credo: The dialectics of one-person and two-person psychologies. *Contemporary Psychoanalysis, 25*, 169–211.

Griffen, F. (2016). *Creative listening and the analytic process*. London: Routledge.

Jung, C. (1969). https://jungcurrents.com.

Knoblauch, S. (2018). Chapter Six: Patterning and linking. In R. Barsness (Ed.), *Core competencies in relational psychoanalysis a guide to practice, study, and research* (p. 142). London: Routledge.

Lester, J. (2005). (Day of Tears – goodreads.com).

Maroda, K. (1998). Enactment: When the patient and the analyst's pasts converge. *Psychoanalytic Psychology, 15*, 517–535.

Maroda, K. (2018). Chapter Nine: Repetition and working through. In R. Barsness (Ed.), *Core competencies in relational psychoanalysis a guide to practice, study, and research* (pp. 87–103). London: Routledge.

McDougall, J. (1980). *A plea for a measure of abnormality*. London. Routledge.

McWilliams, N. (2018). Chapter Five: Therapeutic stance/attitude. In R. Barsness (Ed.), *Core competencies in relational psychoanalysis a guide to practice, study, and research*, (pp. 87–103). London, England: Routledge.

McWilliams, N. (2021). *Psychoanalytic supervision*. New York: Guilford Press.

Michael, J. (2016). (Michael Jr: Know Your Why – YouTube).

Mitchell, S. A. (2000). *Relationality: From attachment to intersubjectivity*. NY. Psychoanalytic Press.

Pizer, S. (2018). Chapter Four: Deep listening/affective attunement. In R. Barsness (Ed.), *Core competencies in relational psychoanalysis a guide to practice, study, and research* (pp. 104–119). London: Routledge.

Schore, A. (2018). Chapter Thirteen: The brain and psychoanalysis. In R. Barsness (Ed.), *Core competencies in relational psychoanalysis a guide to practice, study, and research* (pp. 241–262). London: Routledge.

Shaw, D. (2014). *Traumatic narcissism: Relational systems of subjugation*. London: Routledge.

Shaw, D. (2023). *Analytic love, self-compassion and the growth of internal secure attachment*. Presented to the Chicago Center for Psychoanalysis, October 6, 2023.

Tublin, S. (2018) Chapter Four: Therapeutic intent. In R. Barsness (Ed.), *Core competencies in relational psychoanalysis a guide to practice, study, and research* (pp. 142–157). London: Routledge.

Singer, E. (1970). *Key concepts in psychotherapy*. NY. Basic Books.

Winnicott, D. W. (1949). Mind and its relation to the psyche-soma. In *Through paediatrics to psycho-analysis* (pp. 243–254). London: Hogarth Press.

Winnicott, D. W. (1960). *Playing and reality*. London. Tavistock Publications

# 4    The Essential I

## The Essential I: Presence and the Subjectivity of the Therapist

In Chapter 2, I spoke of the therapist's subjectivity as a critical turn in psychoanalytic theory. This turn shifted our understanding of what constitutes change, namely, that change occurs with two minds (therapist and patient) intersecting, in juxtaposition to one mind (the analyst) analyzing the mind of another (the patient). Jessica Benjamin (2018) describes this psychic process in terms of "the interpenetration of [two] minds, conscious and unconscious, mirror neuron to mirror neuron" (p. 1). This shift sparks in us as clinicians to consider how our subjectivity interpenetrates with our patient's subjectivity and to continually be developing ourselves and our clinical wisdom, as we step out of a stance of objective knowing and into the space of intersubjective play.

To describe what is meant by the use of the therapist's subjectivity the term Essential I is used as a form of expression that emerged in the development of the Certificate Program in Relational Psychodynamic Therapy at the Contemporary Psychodynamic Institute. The term captures the idea of the therapist's subjectivity and calls forth the essentialness of the therapist's presence when conducting psychotherapy.

In preparing to launch the certificate program in relational psychodynamic therapy (RPT), I conducted an Intensive Training and Supervision program for seasoned clinicians, to become Trainer/Supervisors in the Certificate Program. I quickly recognized the absence of the therapists' use of themselves in thinking and working with their patients. Though each of them expressed that their affect was being roused by their patient's story, they tended to downplay their experience. This was particularly true if they were aggressively or erotically aroused. In those highly affective moments, the therapist would dissociate and defer the experience to a countertransference problem, rather than consider the possibility that the experience they may be having is a possible means of the patient trying to make contact. I am sure this has to do with the long tradition we have in the field of negating countertransference experiences rather than using countertransference as a portal or a possible signal that our felt experiences are unique to this particular relationship.

DOI: 10.4324/9781003532828-4

I brought to their attention the unfortunate erasure of the therapist's felt experiences as a means of understanding the other. I drew their attention to Christopher Bollas' (1987) statement that in "order to find the patient, we must look for [them] within ourselves" (p. 202), inferring that we must feel the patient within our own bodies. I mentioned Jessica Benjamins (2018) definition of intersubjectivity as a "relationship of mutual recognition – a relation in which each person experiences the other as a 'like subject,' another mind who can be 'felt with,' yet has a distinct, separate center of feeling and perception" (p. 51) and Lew Arons (2000) comment that we need another mind, in order to find out own (p. 175). I shared with them that the body "speaks," and we must listen to our bodily affective experiences. I indicated to them that the patient consciously and unconsciously wishes to (and can only) reach us through our experiences of them—both mind *and* body. I suggested to these clinicians that though the feelings and experiences the therapist has touches directly upon their own personal subjectivity, these feelings were elicited directly within the therapeutic dyad and thus important to explore. Lew Aron's (1991) words were again helpful. He says,

Patients seek to connect to their analyst, to know them, to probe beneath their professional façade.... much in the same way that children seek to connect and penetrate their parents' inner worlds. The exploration of the patient's experience of the analyst's subjectivity represents one underemphasized aspect of the analysis of transference, and it is an essential aspect of a detailed and thorough explication and articulation of the therapeutic relationship.

(p. 29)

As I continued to emphasize the importance of attending to their own bodily, affective, and countertransference experiences and to track and consider how these affective states consciously and unconsciously are the essence of a relational approach to psychotherapy, there was a collective sigh of relief. The invitation to move out of their heads and into their own affect was not only experienced as relief but also expanded their skill set with working with their patients. They felt invited into working within the "flow of experience; organic-like momentum [relying] on the recognition that each therapist's own subjectivity is affecting the interaction" (Hoffman, 1983, p. 389).

As we grew together in further understanding this important aspect of treatment, and as cases would be presented, we would often end up laughing together at how hard it was to stay connected to our bodily/affective selves in our attempts to understand our patient. This was particularly discovered when they attempted to articulate their affective experiences to the patient. In articulation, the emotion was sucked out of them, offering in its stead, emotionless, cognitive responses. I do not recall who or when but one day we started referring to the self of the therapist as the Essential I. As these clinicians were growing their own sense of agency and challenging their colleagues to do the same, crying out, "where is your \*#\*& "I"," they were beginning to see how essential their presence is to therapeutic success.

I have a friend who is quite the character is provocative, emotional, sassy. She recently told me of her (former) therapist, who she was quite certain hated her. From my friend's point of view, she and the therapist would get caught up in all sorts of emotionally charged entanglements, but when my friend would ask the therapist about what she, the therapist, felt my friend was met with neutral responses. She sensed that the therapist was feigning kindness and understanding rather than engaging her authentically. As the emotional tensions heightened, finally in desperation, my friend said to the therapist, "y'know there are two people in this room and you are not one of them." She then terminated her work with her. Knowing my friend as I do, she would be quite the challenge, but in reporting her experience she said, "there was no there, there." Patients need to know we can be pierced, that we can feel, react and engage in the multiple and complex affective states, including the negative, frightful states that are aroused and to honestly and authentically talk together about these multiple self-states. Gianpiero Petriglieri (2020) states,

> it's easier being in each other's presence, or in each other's
> absence than in the constant presence of each other's absence.

It is not unusual in our practices where two people can gather in a room, and no one is present. Too much therapy is conducted "in the constant presence of each other's absence." The challenge in working relationally and dynamically is that at its core, one must "show up."

Early in my career, challenged by the people with whom I was working, was that to be successful in my career, I would have to show up.

"Moonias! Moonias!" ("White Man! White Man") the children screeched as I stood outside their home on the Maskwacis First Nations Reservation. As a Community Social Worker, I had been summoned to investigate a child abuse allegation. I was twenty-two years old, and it had never occurred to me that the color of my skin was the "thing" determining whether or not I would gain access to this home. The color of my skin "spoke." It spoke of power and the potential to determine the future of this family. I certainly did not have language at the time for what was happening, I only knew what I felt. I felt othered, misunderstood, frightened, alone, even mistreated. Over time, it became clear to me that on the other side of the door was a family that felt the same. At the threshold of our vast differences lay the question: "What will we do with (or to) the other, should the door open?"

I waited.

As I waited, flashing through my mind was the question, "Should I use my state-commissioned authority to enter without their permission or should I wait until the door opened and I was invited in?" And if the door opens, I pondered, "should I exercise my authority to remove the children with no questions asked and get the hell out," or "should I stay, ask questions, and create conversations and together collaborate a plan for the care of these children?"

The door opened and our story began. We would spend the next two years together navigating our differences. As I continued to return, one day I noticed I did not hear the voices of the children yelling "moonias, moonias." Rather, it was the children themselves who opened the door and let me in. Slowly we had moved from Moonias-Indian (First Nations) to the use of our given names. And we became friends. Though I lived ten miles away—when their parents would sit for hours in the bar, leaving the children in the car or on the streets, these three siblings eventually found where I lived and I have the mixed memory or sadness and madness, with the joy of them sitting at the table over a can of Campbell's soup and grilled cheese that I made for us.

One morning, I received a message from the police that the children of this family were sitting in a cell at the police station waiting for me to take them home. The children had we apprehended by the police for breaking into several stores and were sitting at the police station and they had been unsuccessful in contacting their mother or any other family member. The children had directed the police to call me. As we drove back toward the reservation one of the children spoke up and said, "Roy, if you would come see us more often, we would be better." The words struck deep. And they have never left me. That small child, speaking from deep within their heart, was very wise. For we are all made better when someone shows up.

Perhaps because of my youth, my idealism, if I did nothing else, I returned. But my confidence in continuing to return was because the Maskwacis slowly welcomed my return. Their acceptance of me as the White man that I am, challenged me to accept them, as the persons that they are. It was they who initiated in me that, "to be useful in this world, the best I can do is to be me and not try to be you or attempt to make you me." This was a challenge to my previous gross understanding where difference was expected to accommodate my whiteness. What I have learned is that it is in the grit of working through difference, misunderstandings, misrecognitions, ruptures, and repairs—where transformation takes place.

I have been a decades long student of the philosopher Martin Buber whose work entitled: I/Thou is a classic. A quick read of Buber often leaves the reader thinking the I/Thou encounter is simply a moment of meeting when two persons come to understand the other and tension is released. But the I/Thou moment is not encountered through sameness, agreement, or compromise. Rather, it is predicated on the recognition of difference. Genuine Encounter is the act of living in the ache and the beauty of contrast. It is the move from using the other as an object for personal gain and power. It is the act of turning toward the other as a sacred other. It is the hope that two separates can find unity in contrast.

This is not achievable however, if one is unable to confirm oneself. If one is unable to live and be in their own skin—(in my case, my white skin)—the skin of the stranger will always be someone to fear, to subjugate, to own and objectify. But if I am able to consider my fear of the other as an outward manifestation of unworked issues of my own, at the least this should give me pause toward an understanding of the other as an unfair recipient of my biases. At the most, it should cause me to turn toward the other with humility, with wonder and with awe.

One must be located within themselves—their own traditions, culture, aches and pains of their own humanity, in order to be dislocated, upended through the genuine encounter with another—in order to be relocated into a new and more vital experience. Brenda's request was specific. It was a specific call to me. She said, ROY, if YOU. She was calling me out. She wasn't calling for a Social Worker, she was calling for me, Roy. When people seek our help, they specifically call us to be present.

As I moved on to further study and eventually to becoming a psychologist, my first patient again reminded me of the importance of showing up. Swept up in curing and fixing, as a novice in my very first practicum, I would try anything and everything that I learned in class and then the very next day try it out on my unassuming patients. My first patient assigned to me put up with my antics for a time. But when I brought in a huge piece of paper, and multi-colored pens and stood standing with my 6'2" frame looming over her pronouncing that today our assignment was to complete the genogram, she gently and quite courageously said, "put that a way and when you are ready to hear my story, I will tell you." I was stunned and as I put the material aside, I sat down, and I knew that my work as a psychologist was about to change rather drastically. I sensed at that moment that what happens between two people in the context of a therapy relationship had truly little to do with insight or fixing. Rather, what it would require of me was to risk living into the uncharted waters of the patient's narrative, listening to their story as it stirs and stews in my own body and mind, in order for the patient to discover the lost and hidden parts of their story that is troubling them.

These wise teachers of mine introduced me to a therapeutic awareness that to help others requires a radical openness to oneself, my own vulnerabilities, thoughts, affects in order to be open and available to the other. Change, I learned, would come, not through my well thought out, perfectly timed interpretations or wisdom but through suffering with (withness). And to be with another, I discovered, requires that I am able to be with myself.

Show up, show up show up—these wise ones said, because when you show up, I will find my way to do the same. To show up we must have an awareness and acceptance of our own human condition, our strengths, our flaws, our fears, our shame, and frankly, a humility that connects with the challenge of simply being human to understand our patients.

A common refrain that has been around too long in our education is the idea that we can only take our patients as far as we have been healed ourselves. Though there is some wisdom in this statement, the problem with the statement is that it robs the therapist of their ongoing growth as a person and infers that healing is finite. Our expertise is not always connected to how healed we are. Many times, we enter a session broken. And just as we try to help our patients work through their pain and suffering, we can do so only if we are fully alive to our own. A patient once said to me, "I envy you because you have it all figured out." To which I replied, "that is not true. And if it were true, I would not be of much help to you." I continued, "I don't think we are here to get" figured out. I think we are here trying to figure out how to live fully in all the pain and the joys of being human. To help you, I must be fully living my life as fully as I can as well.

While our expertise undoubtedly relies on maintaining a robust level of mental health and well-being, it is crucial to acknowledge our shared humanity. Our true expertise lies in our ability to authentically engage with our own journey of growth and transformation. Personally, I've found that many of my patients have surpassed me in their own journey toward growth.

To articulate this concept, I often draw upon Winnicott's depiction of the True Self not as a fixed entity, but as an ineffable aspect of existence that eludes complete understanding, both by ourselves and others. It serves as the wellspring of spontaneous expression, continuously unfolding within us. At the heart of this Essential Self lies not perfection, but rather an innate sense of being, characterized by grace, humility, spontaneity, and a profound openness to both self and others.

The vocational call to becoming a therapist is both noble and self-serving. People enter this field because they want to help others—but they are also seeking ways to understand themselves. Long before we enter training, we are already analysts of our own souls, trying to figure ourselves out in relationship to significant others in our lives and to our place in the world.

This inborn interest and drive to know is the gift we bring to the therapeutic encounter. However, this quest for human growth is riddled with fear and anxiety and is often shrouded in conflict avoidance and shame. And most people attracted to this field tend to be conflict avoidant and are just as prone to low self-esteem and shame as the persons who seek their assistance. Though the research on positive therapeutic outcome is conditioned upon the richness of connectedness between the therapist and the patient, therapy often slopes toward disconnection. Why? Because the therapists' own self-value is compromised and connectedness to another, is complicated. Consequently, the very thing that can heal—therapist/patient connectedness—is often forfeited, replaced with pseudo-empathy, advice giving, behavioral interventions and any other tools that keep the therapist safe from the inevitable entanglements of authentic relating.

The Essential I is directly related to our self-esteem. Nancy McWilliams (2021) says,

> Self-esteem that is realistic reflects reasonable (i.e. neither perfectionistic nor falsely inflated) criterion for self-evaluation. Self-esteem that is reliable protects against being devastated by criticism or manipulated by adulation. It allows us to evaluate negative feedback without collapsing

internally and positive feedback without being seduced by flattery. Healthy self-esteem comes from internalizing caregivers' non-shaming attitudes toward our authentic feelings, thoughts and behaviors.

(p. 56)

Philosopher Martin Buber (2015) writes, "every person born into this world represents something new, something that never existed before, something original and unique" (p. 66).

In the same spirit, Rabbi Zusya asks himself, "in the world to come I shall not be asked: "why were you not Moses?" I shall be asked, "why were you not Zusya?"

The word "hakomi" from the Hopi Nation asks, "how do I stand in relation to these many realms?" It is this question that every therapist must answer before becoming a clinician. Our first question is not, who is this person/patient before me but, "who am I?" in relation to myself and to the other.

Winnicott's idea of the true self emerged from his observation of his students whom he saw as remarkably frightened into conformity His wish for them was that they would not simply be imitations of others but come into their own sense of worth, valuing their own mind and possessing confidence in the expression of their own viewpoints.

Bryan Nixon (2020, personal communication) a Trainer in the RPT program at the Contemporary Psychodynamic Institute offers his own reflection on his own Essential I and says,

> I want to orient my life in such a way that the end of my life will permit me to smile and exhale with gratitude. I want to embrace my eventual death now, as fully as possible, so that I do not dread it when it is upon me. I believe this will offer me the greatest gift – to be my most authentic self in the here and now, to be able to frolic in the conflicts of life as they arise within myself, with my spouse, my children, with my friends and in my work in this world. I am committed to the belief that as I bring my Essential "I" to the world that the world will be a better place.

Within RPT we speak of the Essential "I" for the potential space of "We." Implicit in that statement is that in order to help another, the person of the therapist must receive the totality of his or her own self. This includes "a healthy narcissism, which functions as a protection against becoming a martyr as a therapist." The Essential I recognizes that I, as the therapist, matter too, and it isn't helpful for either the therapist or the patient to stay in a position of containing and accepting or allowing dynamics that challenge the therapeutic frame.

It is from this "I" that we can bring a deeper curiosity and presence to situations where, for example, we might have turned a blind eye to an unpaid balance, extended sessions, or a silent tolerance of harassment or aggression towards the therapist.

It is from this "I" that we can ask ourselves and the patient questions like, "how is it ok for you to talk to me like that?" It is from this I that we can ask ourselves and the patient, "What the hell is going on here anyway?" thereby getting deeper into an experiential understanding of what is occurring in the relational dyad. It is also the place where we can set boundaries around what is necessary for the work to occur (payment of fees, no harassment or threats of therapist, etc. (Clarissa Hill, 2024, Personal Communication). To work from a relationally psychodynamic perspective, the therapist must have a particularly good sense of their "I-amness" for the patient to discover their own. The "I" almost precedes the "we."

In South Africa, the Zulu greeting "Sawubona" is widely used. This greeting is accompanied by a respectful nod and means "I see you." It is a way of acknowledging the presence and worth of the person being greeted. In response, one would say "Ngikhona," which means "I am here." This exchange of greetings establishes a connection and builds a sense of unity.

The question, "where are you?" is a question that positions itself whenever we gather with our patients (and within our world). Can you answer, I am here!?

## Radical Openness

When contemporary psychoanalytic thinking, shifted the nucleus of the analytic relationship from the analyst as neutral observer/container/knower to an active subject where both the patient and the analyst are activated to participate within the narrative of the patient's story, a new level of self-reflection was ushered in. Working within a relational psychodynamic model, the self of the therapist is far more exposed than the psychoanalyst of the past. No longer protected by the luxury of anonymity, we are left with a greater responsibility of becoming radically open to our own subjectivity within the therapeutic dyad. When we can answer the question, "where are you?" and say, "I am here," introduces the potential of listening to our patients from within our own inner experience of them.

Dr. Anton Harts article *Multicultural Competence and Radical Openness* (2017), identifies himself as

> multiracial, with a black father whose ancestors were African American, Native American and Western European, and a white, Jewish mother whose ancestors were from Russia and Poland. He says, I consider myself to be both black and white, and also not simply either.
>
> (p. 27)

I share the richness of Dr. Hart's self-identification as it speaks not only of his multiracial identity but also of the complexity and the multiplicity of the human condition. It also challenges all of us to consider our own complexity, the complexity of our patients, and invites each of us to be radically open to our multiple, complex selves and toward others.

Dr. Hart (2017) is a relational psychoanalyst and though the article mentioned above speaks to race and relational psychoanalysis, the article powerfully addresses a stance of radical openness to each of us in all contexts of our lives and how we position ourselves with our patients and in the world. He states,

> The heart of the matter is learning how to become increasingly undefended around matters of diversity and otherness such that you can be open: open to the other person who will be in some significant ways, most certainly different from you. A psychoanalytic sensibility suggests to us that genuine openness can only emerge in the context of an unscripted dialogue, one that involves making contact with and participating in an exchange that will, necessarily, threaten the dialogic participants' understandings, identities and perceptions.
>
> (p. 12)

Though, the use of the therapist's inner experience of their patient is hinted upon throughout psychoanalysis, the therapeutic process itself, has most often steered its attention toward the analysis of the patient's inner workings without due processing of the analyst's self-experience. However, since the inception of psychoanalytic theory, Freud (1953) recognized the highly subjective nature of the therapeutic experience, stating, "No one who, like me, conjures up the most evil of those half-tamed demons that inhabit the human beast and seeks to wrestle with them, can expect to come through the struggle unscathed" (p. 45). Theodor Reik in 1948 wrote an important text entitled: *Listening with the Third Year: the inner experience of a psychoanalyst,* and states,

> when our ears are properly attuned and we are listening well, the shards of memory and imagination that arise from within constitute meaningful and often illuminating responses to our patients' communications. Such experiences have taught us that our ability to understand another person depends on our capacity, not only to listen to that individual, but to ourselves as well. And we have learned something else: that *among the tools of the analyst's trade none is more valuable than the effective use of himself* [italics mine].
>
> (p. 145)

Jessica Benjamin (2018) observes that intersubjective theory thrusts the analyst into the non-linear system of two subjects, each capable of destabilizing the other's self-certainty at any moment, leading to emergent meanings (p. 3). In the context of relational theory, where the subjectivity of the therapist is integral to the therapeutic process, the therapist becomes more vulnerable than the psychoanalyst of the past.

Working intersubjectively may initially seem daunting, appearing to demand a significant emotional investment from the therapist. However, the reality is quite the opposite. Affect states, unconscious communications, interpersonal actions, and reactions are inherently present from the very first meeting. Denying these various self-states through intellectualization and objectivity is counterintuitive, counterproductive, and requires greater effort. By immersing oneself in the experience, attending to the therapist's own deep affective states elicited by the patient, and actively engaging in the discovery of what is happening, the treatment remains vibrant. Ignoring what is in the foreground dulls the therapeutic space. The therapist's subjectivity is always present, and the key question is how best to work with it.

Ultimately, by turning our affective experiences with patients inward and exploring our own emotional responses, we gain insight into the patient's internal struggles and the dynamics of the therapeutic relationship.

Entering the therapist's subjectivity into the treatment is a formidable task, requiring a realistic and radical openness to countertransference issues, a stable self-esteem, a shift from a protective interpretive stance to analyzing the therapeutic dyad, affective attunement, a deep consideration of unconscious manifestations within the therapist and the patient, conflict resolution within the therapeutic dialogue, tolerance of contrast, appreciation for the patient's experience of the therapist, and the recognition of the value of surrendering certainty through co-metabolization.

Working from a relational psychodynamic model does indeed threaten the security of our typical empathic, nurturing professional selves as well as our identities and self-perceptions. It also challenges our tendency to avoid conflict. But part of understanding the "essential" in the Essential I, is that for us to work relationally, it is "essential" that we are willing to be radically open to ourselves and confront our fears and self-protective defenses.

Radical openness is generally thought of as a particular stance we hold toward our patients. This stance, however, is a bit of an illusion and compromises authenticity. Of course, we must provide a safe place, but safety must still allow for difference. Safe does not mean that we enter the relationship without prejudice and judgment. In fact, if we seek to withhold our prejudices and judgment, authenticity is immediately compromised. A stance of radical openness represents a dialogic space where the patient *and* the therapist attempt to meet one another honestly and to speak to that which often threatens our security and working out together our prejudices, judgments, conflicts, and differences, inherent in any authentic relationship. A fundamental aspect of the relational psychodynamic approach is the therapist's receptivity to the patient's experiences and feedback. This openness enables the therapist to reflect on how their own subjectivity influences the patient. Such a perspective extends beyond the confines of therapy into our broader societal roles. Embracing a dialogical way of thinking, practicing, and living can transform our interactions, not just in therapy, but across cultural, political, religious domains, and in the authenticity with which we engage every facet of life.

Therapists are a unique breed. We are thin-skinned people, affectively permeable and intuitive. We live close to our hearts. This is good. Until it isn't.

When aspects of ourselves get revealed, we tend to overly personalize our feelings and more dangerously disavow them. We do this by placing them outside of ourselves and into the person with whom we feel threatened, including our patients. This is so commonly done in psychotherapy through the convenience of pathologizing our patients, we don't even notice it. Radical openness toward our own pathologies and countertransference reactions assists us in breaking through a defensive posture that disavows or disengages and projects onto our patients unwanted affective states, insecurities, often locating them in the other.

Most therapists prefer to be perceived as the good object. Furthermore, we are hard-wired to defend when negative aspects of ourselves become revealed. To work from a relational perspective challenges us in our own personal lives often breaking open those unwanted self-states we have hidden. And yet, "a psychoanalytic sensibility...that threaten the dialogic participants' understandings, identities and perceptions" is the impetus for change" (Hart, 2017, p. 12). In the breaking open, the therapists' emotional states were expanded, they had a deeper awareness and concern for their patient and their defensiveness toward themselves and their patient, became useful for further analytic dialogue. Poet Rosemerry Wahtola Trommer (2018) in her poem, *The Way It Is*, speaks of breaking open in this way,

> Over and over we break
> open, we break and
> we break and we open.
> For a while, we try to fix
> the vessel – as if
> to be broken is bad.
> As if with glue and tape
> and a steady hand we
> might bring things to perfect
> again. As if they were ever
> perfect. As if to be broken is not
> also perfect. As if to be open
> is not the path toward joy.
> The vase that's been shattered
> and cracked will never
> hold water. Eventually
> it will leak. And at some point,
> perhaps, we decide
> that we're done with picking
> our flowers anyway, and no
> longer need a place to contain them.
> We watch them grow just
> as wildflowers do – unfenced,
> unmanaged, blossoming only

when they're ready – and my god,
how beautiful they are amidst
the mounting pile of shards.

Breaking open the therapist's own subjectivity (radical openness) comes with a risk and threatens our well-crafted security which we often seek to deny or quell. But holding to a genuine stance of inquiry and staying and working through the conflicts, the risk of doing so is most always generative. Hart (2017) continues,

> If we can stand to stay in the conversation (and encourage our dialogic others to do so as well), we may…be able to relinquish…the self-protective blindness and biases we contain in favor of novel ways of people seeing and being with difference.

(p. 27)

By pursuing a radical openness toward our own subjective affective states initiated directly in relationship to our patients and to our countertransference reactions, therapeutic space is vitalized. Being in the presence of a therapist, open to their inner experience in relation to their patient, gives room for the patient to also risk a radical openness to their own life. And breaking open is good for us all and is at the heart of a good analysis. The I that treats the other as an object to be analyzed is an I that cannot grow or mature. In contrast, the Essential I approaches themselves and other as subject and in so doing, growth of both persons is attained.

## References

Aron, L. (1991). The patient's experience of the analyst's subjectivity. *Psychoanalytic Dialogues*, 1(1), 29–51.

Aron, L. (2000). *A meeting of minds: Mutuality in psychoanalysis*. Routledge.

Benjamin, J. (2018). *Beyond doer and done to: Recognition theory, intersubjectivity, and the Third*. London: Routledge.

Bollas, C. (1987). *The shadow of the object: Psychoanalysis of the unthought known*. New York: Columbia University Press.

Buber, M. (2015). *Hasidism and modern man*. Princeton, NJ: Princeton University Press.

Freud, S. (1953). Fragment of an analysis of a case of hysteria. *Standard Edition*, 7, 3–122. London: Hogarth Press.

Hart, A. (2017). Multicultural competence to radical openness. *The American Psychoanalyst*, 51, 12–13, 26–27.

Hill, C. (2024). Personal communication.

Hoffman, I. Z. (1983). The patient as interpreter of the analyst's experience. *Contemporary Psychoanalysis*, 19, 389–423.

McWilliams, N. (2021). *Psychoanalytic supervision*. New York: Guilford Press.

Nixon, B. (2020). *Comprehensive handbook for contemporary psychodynamic institute*. Seattle, WA. CPI Publications.

Petriglieri, G. (2020, April 13). The psychology behind effective remote teams. *Harvard Business Review*. https://hbr.org/2020/04/the-psychology-behind-effective-remote-teams

Reik, T. (1948). *Listening with the third ear: The inner experience of a psychoanalyst*. New York: Farrar, Straus & Co.

Trommer, R. W. (2018). *The way it is*. San Jose, CA: Able Muse Press.

# The MAMAL Method

**PART ONE: AN INTRODUCTION**

Let's take a moment to recap where we have come from and where we are headed. So far, I have presented an overview of the theoretical foundations in the practice of relational psychodynamic therapy (RPT) (Chapter 2) and a review of the text *Core Competencies in Relational Psychoanalysis: A Guide to Practice, Study, and Research* (Chapter 3). Then I introduced the concept of the use of the therapist's subjectivity in psychotherapy and the idea of Radical Openness—a therapeutic stance not only toward our patients but also equally essential, a radical openness toward the therapist's own subjectivity (Chapter 4).

Chapter 5 now takes us inside the consultation room where I will present to you the MAMAL method of supervision. The M in the MAMAL acronym represents the muse, A—affect, M—metabolization, A—articulation, and L—learning. I will speak to each of these areas separately in this chapter. It's important to note that this model is dynamic, not linear. We're always musing, engaging affectively, metabolizing, articulating, and learning throughout the entire MAMAL process. The primary goal of relational psychodynamic supervision is to develop the clinical skills of affect, metabolization, and articulation and for members to grow in their experience of engaging in intersubjective play.

In the MAMAL method, emphasis is placed upon each member of the group and the supervisor to immerse themselves within the patient's narrative by (1) attending to their own affective arousals and intersubjective experiences in relationship to the presenting case, (2) developing a clinical mind around their experience, and (3) practicing and building relational language. This supervisory stance is a significant shift from the more common supervisory stance that places the primary focus on figuring out the patient or advising the therapist. In contrast, the MAMAL model works at assisting each group member at figuring out their own mind as it is felt in direct relationship to the patient.

In the MAMAL method, the supervisor role is three-fold:

1 **Engagement and Vulnerability**: The supervisor actively engages their own subjectivity within the group process and is fully immersed in the patient's narrative alongside the participants, demonstrating in vivo the MAMAL process. The therapist's vulnerability encourages the vulnerability of the participants and in turn a strong bond between the participants develops. The supervisor does not assume the role of "truth teller," but is an engaged co-participant who facilitates the process by disclosing their own affective experiences, metabolizations, and articulations.

2 **Central Thou**: The supervisor understands that central to all successful learning communities is a clear purpose and a solid leader. They are that leader, serving as the dynamic connector for the group, assisting in integrating clinical practices with theory and teaching and modeling the core tenets of the MAMAL method: (1) the use of the therapist's self and the

importance of presence, (2) the powerful use of multiple affective states, and (3) the courage to speak with honesty, humility, and respect, fostering growth through mutuality and reciprocity. Given the immersive nature of supervision, it is anticipated that supervisors will also at times find themselves disoriented. However, it is their readiness to recognize this possibility, coupled with a commitment to transparency and self-reflection—often conducted openly in front of their supervisees—that allows them to demonstrate the art of metabolization as they consider their thoughts as to what happened, what is happening and how they have become entangled or muddled and how it is related to the case. Group processes also flow through the supervisor, both as full participant as well as the person who sustains a space for genuine encounters to grow among members, aiming to foster genuine cohesion and respect.

3 **Fluency and Lifelong Learning**: The supervisor is proficient in both theory and practice and values lifelong learning. They are committed to their own growth and actively pursue further education and development.

The MAMAL method is a process of discovery, imagination, and co-participation through shared affective experiences in relationship to a particular case. This approach assists the group members (1) to deepen their self-reflective skills in direct response to their experience of the presenting patient, (2) to increase their capacity to metabolize affect, (3) to attune to unconscious urgings, replications, and self-other experiences, (4) to develop articulation skills and confidence in speaking authentically to their patients, and (5) to cultivate confidence working from an intersubjective perspective by engaging in the inevitable repetitions, misunderstandings, and entanglements that occur within psychodynamic psychotherapy.

**PART TWO: THE MUSE**

In the MAMAL method, the presenting case serves as the muse and the source of inspiration for each member to consider and with whom to work. This is in contrast to more common supervision models that concentrate on the patient or the presenter as the primary focus of inquiry. Sophia Richman (2014) conceptualizes the muse as:

> an embodied image of an imaginary other who serves as a mirroring, inspiring, and witnessing function for the artist. Like an imaginary friend, the Muse exists in the intermediate area of experience [to what she refers to as] potential space…it is a relational presence in what would otherwise be a solitary activity of making art.
>
> (p. 3)

The muse in literature and in film is the main character and source of inspiration that sets the stage for the story. The protagonist (muse) moves the story forward, usually in a struggle either against someone or something. Or in response to an existential conflict within themselves. As the readers of the novel or viewers of the film get into the story and play with it, they have reactions, thoughts and feelings, for and against the primary actor (muse).

Think of the Joker in Batman. The Joker is a highly controversial character who captures the viewer's mind and heart by confronting his own existential angst as well as his troubled conflicted relationship with Batman. Fighting the forces of both love and hate, our experience of the Joker arouses multiple affective states from passion to disgust to hatred.

In the MAMAL method, the presenting case becomes the muse, the protagonist, the one to whom each member of the group directs their emotions and their minds. The group supervision begins with the presenting therapist giving a brief summary (around 20 minutes) of their work with their patient (the muse). The organizing question for each member as they listen to the muse is: "How is this patient (the Muse) infecting you?" (Affect) "What are your thoughts as to *what* and *why*?" (Metabolization). One of the portals into metabolizing is to ask: *"What* is this experience trying to tell me?" and *"Why* has this affective experience occurred?" We metabolize not only to find an explanation or to make meaning but also to get deeper into the full narrative of the patient's story. And finally: *"How* do you imagine you would engage your mind and your affects with this patient?" (Articulation).

The supervisor is required to fully immerse themselves in the process modeling for the group their own affective experiences of the muse, demonstrate their work of metabolization and their efforts in articulation. Additionally, the supervisor is responsible for guiding the group in remaining focused on their own affective experiences, steering away from the temptation to supervise the presenter or the presenter's case.

While the instruction to consider the patient as the muse may seem clear and straightforward, it is common for each group member and the supervisor to deviate from their own affective experience of the patient/muse and return their focus to the more common approach of supervising the case presenter or the presenting case itself. This urge to digress is quite strong. The supervisor must maintain the frame and encourage each group member, including themselves, to hold the patient as the muse and to keep metabolizing their own affective experiences. This all-hands-on-deck approach is about growing the reflective capacities of each of the group members' minds by attending to each member's affective experiences, leading to greater metabolization and movement toward the practice of articulation. As the presenter witnesses a diversity of minds and experiences embodied in their group their own mind/experiences about their patient are expanded, as are the clinical minds of each member of the group. Group members will often find themselves commenting in amazement, "When we share our minds with one another, all minds grow!"

Though our traditional supervision models tend to think that a supervisor may know best what to do with a patient, the truth is, the best a supervisor can do is enlarge the therapist's mind about their patient. Therefore, the supervisor and the group members offer their experience of how the patient's narrative, as told by the therapist, "infects" them. By having creative collaborators who allow themselves to participate and imagine the presenter's patient as though it were their own and do not tell the therapist what to do or assume their knowledge of the patient exceeds that of the presenter, this non-authoritarian, radically open, and curious approach offers the therapist (and the collaborators) multiple possibilities in working with this patient. Approaching the case from this perspective, the complexity of the patient's story is thickened, empathy for the patient is deepened, and in the language of "extended cognition" the clinical minds of all group members are "supersized" (Strawn & Brown, 2012).

The purpose of introducing the muse is to ignite the emotions and the intellect of each participant. As group members share their encounters with the muse, their clinical minds are activated and enriched which deepens the complexity of the case. This process resembles an orchestra preparing for a performance where members gather, tuning their instruments amidst chatter and camaraderie, gearing up for the spectacle! Then, as the conductor steps onto the podium and raises their baton, a symphony of diverse instruments harmonizes into a captivating complexity, stirring our senses, our emotions, and our intellect.

**PART THREE: AFFECT**

## The Primacy of Affect: We Find Our Patients through Our Gut

> Words, words, words – and all I can do is **feel**.
> – (thirteen-year-old boy responding to his father's words in effort to
> discipline some errant behavior. The father? Me)

Early in my career, I had the opportunity to read Erwin Singer's text, *Key Concepts in* Psychotherapy (1965). His words had a profound impact on my clinical development which continues to this day. He said:

> Hearing is not to proceed by listening with the ear; a much more pro-
> found listening or hearing is called for, a hearing with the third or inner
> ear, with one's VISCERA (caps mine) with one's full being: an attending
> to one's inner voices…it is total involvement in one's reactions to stimuli
> which is deemed activity.
>
> (p. 64)

The word *viscera* hit me in my gut! For I knew, intuitively, that what I was feeling viscerally, was directly connected to my patient. My training had failed me in teaching me that my expertise was in my capacity in providing precise and detailed assessment, diagnosis, formulations, and clever inter-pretations. Attention to my bodily experience as a critical aspect with which to help my patients was not considered. In fact, in most training, one's emo-tions are expected to be cautiously guarded as countertransference issues and placed outside the consulting room. When I read Singer on that day, I can almost say that there was rejoicing. A permission to use what I had in-tuitively felt all along.

I did not think too much about who Erwin Singer might be as I read him on that day or continued to teach his insight in my classroom. Furthermore, despite his spirited writing I held a stereotype of him as a guarded, neutral Freudian analyst. Recently, I decided to find out more about who he was, and my stereotype was shattered.

What I learned was that Erwin Singer (1919–1980) was a vibrant, labyrin-thian human being. Edgar Levenson described him as Rabelaisian—earthy, vigorous, lively, irreverent. He says:

> Erwin took authentic risks in therapy. When they worked, they worked,
> and when they failed, they failed. He knew the dangers and wrote about
> them, but he preferred a genuine mistake to a craven beyond-the-couch
> apathy or boredom. None ever said of Erwin, as did the patient in *Port-
> noy's Complaint* of her therapist, "I know he must be alive, I can hear
> him breathing." No, Levenson continues, "with Erwin, you could hear
> him living."
>
> (in Natchez, 1982, p. 304)

Gladys Natchez (1982), another friend who gave tribute to Singer at his memorial, said,

> He was a multidimensional man an actor, skier.... sommelier...fighter for political freedom...possessing vitality, charisma, lustiness, gusto, fullness and love of life!
>
> (p. 304)

I believe the following words of Singer would have been a fine benediction at his own memorial service. He wrote,

"Always live. Just live, with all the agony and the ecstasy that it brings. Just live!"

A tragedy that he only lived for 61 years. But we get a sense he lived! May this be true for all of us who practice this sacred art of psychotherapy by attending to our viscera in our work.

Psychiatric problems are emotional problems; they are problems in affect integration caused by failures in attunement and reciprocity. Emotion is the primary conduit for transformation and when engaged and worked through brings healing and lasting change. The reason people come to treatment is not to improve their mind by changing their thinking, but to change their mind by connecting to their split-off emotions embedded within their unconscious. This requires the psychodynamic therapist to listen to what is beneath the words of the patient's story. We do so by attending to our viscera. It is our affective experiences which vitalize our work, connect us to our patient's intra/interpersonal world, and bring us into the risky space of intersubjective play.

Through affective states, we recognize what is stimulated within the therapist is, in part, a transmission of the patient's internal and external world, yet unknown or unspoken. Therefore, the psychodynamic listener seeks to be permeable allowing another person's story to "get under their skin" and into their hearts and their minds. The therapist gains access to the patient through their affective experience awakened within them vis a viz their patient.

Theodor Reik called this specialized listening as listening with "the third ear," Thomas Ogden, calls it "reverie." I have referred to listening as listening to the "conversation that is at hand." A type of listening that listens for the unspeakable seeking voice. As noted above, Singer talks about listening with the third or inner ear, with one's full being [with full] involvement in one's reactions to stimuli. Such activity requires utmost effort (Singer, 1965, p. 58). To understand the patient the therapist must be able to be "infected" by their emotional world.

Research in the neurosciences supports this idea as it continues to discover that the emotional brain–right-brain to right-brain communications, those affective states and interactions "beneath the words," (Schore, 2018, p. 246) oscillating between the therapist and the patient (intersubjectivity) is essential for affect regulation and the development of the neo-cortex. The neo-cortex is the part of the brain that regulates, reasons, reflects, and gives language to emotion. The more therapists facilitate deep affective experiences, the greater likelihood of more positive outcomes.

Schore (2018) goes on to say that it is in "heightened affective moments [where] the patient's unconscious internal working model of attachment, whether secure or insecure, is reactivated…and re-enacted in the psychotherapeutic relationship [where change takes place]" (p. 245). Relational conflict has a way of getting us to a deep emotional level. Conflict wakes us up! It gets our hearts racing and our minds going.

Additionally, our bodies are hard-wired to feel before we think. For example, when we experience fear or relational trauma, we feel it in our body first. In response to stress, the body's sympathetic nervous system is activated by a sudden release of hormones stimulated by our adrenal glands. A deep physiological reaction occurs when we are in the presence of something or someone we fear.

From early attachment theory to present day research on emotion (Ainsworth, Bowlby, Schore, Siegel, Porges, Fosha), we know that psychological well-being and optimal brain growth, are dependent upon attuned, resonant dyadic interactions. We also know that repair of ruptures in misattunement leads to further emotional growth and development. Therefore, therapies that prioritize affect and constructive conflict within the therapeutic relationship are the therapies most likely to impart long-term shifts in affective regulation and emotional well-being.

Unfortunately, early psychoanalytic theory viewed therapists' affective experiences as countertransference reactions and viewed countertransference as interference and consequently kept from analytic investigation. Negative countertransference reactions were considered a defense projected onto the therapist by the patient and meant to be interpreted rather than perceived as a means of communication. This stance stifled the power and potential usefulness of the use of countertransference. In contemporary models, the therapist's affective experiences are seen as critical to the development of affect integration and optimal growth of the brain. By attending to the impact of the patient's life on the viscera of the therapist, the patient has in real time an authentic affective experience of the impact of their story on their therapist.

The uniqueness of the relational approach is the movement away from a blank screen interpretive model toward direct involvement in the emotional field of the therapist/patient interaction. When we practice from what is known as a two-person psychology, the therapist's affective states, in relation to the patient's affective states, take center stage in the work. As the therapist shifts their attention from cognitive formulations down to their viscera, they gain access to the deep affective states of their patient.

In relational psychodynamic supervision using the MAMAL method, it is important for the supervisor to guide group members in locating their affect and reflecting upon their various affective states in relation to the patient's state of mind, their past, and the patients' affective states. This getting a "feel" for the patient comes by attending to the feelings made present in the therapist.

## No Affect

It is common in supervision to hear someone say they have no feelings. They often report this as feeling bored—to which I find myself responding, "That is a feeling!" Often it is the patient who is cast as the boring one! This is an error and an unfortunate one. For though the patient may not be the most interesting one of the day, when we probe the therapist's absence of affective experience, it is almost always because the therapist has also checked out. When we push in further, we find a defensive reason for why the therapist has lost their affective experiences. When there is no feeling, we need to check what affect state we may be dissociating and bring the affective state to the patient. We do this by considering together our thoughts about why and how this is occurring. Though it may feel uncomfortable, it is the responsibility of the therapist to bring attention to the no-affect dilemma both within themselves and with their patient.

## Empathy/Authenticity

A fundamental expectation of most models of treatment is that the therapist provides a safe and empathic space for their patients. Though there may be varied understandings of the term, therapists often confuse empathy with "being nice [rather] than with being useful" (Klein, Bernard, & Schermer, 2010, p. 30). Maroda (2021) states,

> If one accepts that emotion is the currency of therapeutic action, then it is incumbent upon us to deal more directly with the emotion that flows through the analytic dyad. Doing so requires a high level of self-awareness in the analyst, requiring the aforementioned relinquishment of our claims on "goodness" in favor of authenticity.
>
> (p. 202)

Neuroscience researcher Louis Cozolino (2010) states the human brain is not a "static organ," (p. 19) it's a "social organ" (p. 12). "Emotionally stimulating interactions [with other human persons] generate brain growth" (Cozolino, 2006, p. 86). "Without mutually stimulating interactions, people and neurons wither and die…From birth until death, each of us needs others who seek us out, [and] show interest in discovering who we are" (Cozolino, 2006, p. 11). Since the human brain is "experience dependent" and shaped and reshaped by experiences, a genuine *authentic* relational encounter with another human being changes the chemistry and structure of the brain.

When our patients come to see us, they want more than just our clinical minds. They are looking for an authentic response from us. They want to know how they are experienced. Courageous speech discipline spontaneity is: "Do I have the courage to bring my experience to them?" And though the patient's safety always remains essential, attempting to apply an empathic space, void of authenticity, gets in the way of an effective treatment.

Empathy within psychoanalysis became a topic in the 1970s through the work of Heinz Kohut. In his book, *The Analysis of the* Self (1970) Kohut explores the idea of self-love (narcissism) suggesting that some level of narcissism was healthy and that if persons experienced sufficient mirroring (empathy) alongside optimal frustration, the capacity to love oneself and others was made possible. In contrast to the Freudian drive theory as the primary organization of the psyche, Kohut came to believe that at the root of psychological discontent and disorganization of the psyche, was a failure in empathic attunement. The failure to provide empathy resulted in low self-esteem and shame.

Disorders of the self, according to Kohut, are manifested by the wish to perceive others as an extension of themselves (mirror transference); to idealize others with whom they can merge (idealized object); or to imitate others in order to achieve a sense of self-worth (twinship transference). The analyst's task is to provide sufficient empathic interest that permits the natural reoccurrence of these three different transferences to be re-experienced and through empathic attunement the analyst serves as a corrective emotional experience for the patient. Kohut's theory is deeply entrenched within psychoanalysis today, and any new student to the field will be taught that their fundamental task is to adopt an empathic stance toward their patients and to provide a corrective emotional experience for the patient.

However, Bolognini (1997) who has studied empathy over the past thirty years, takes issue with Kohut's view of empathy, particularly, empathy as something the therapist can apply or in his own words, "an all-purpose instrument to be deployed at will" (p. 279). Applied empathy (empathism) becomes a dogma, a technique that implies "doing" empathy will create change.

Physician Jane Macnaughton (2009) in her article: *The Dangerous Practice of Empathy*, suggests that we recomplicate the word. Her concern is "that empathy has become an act – something we think about doing or providing for the patient, rather than attending to what is aroused within our sub-cortical brainstem where we feel the patient before we can think of them" (p. 40). She uses an example of medical schools using a teaching tool with the acronym E.M.P.A.T.H.Y. developed by Helen Riess at empathetics.com. The acronym stands for eye contact, muscles of facial expression, posture, affect, tone of voice, hearing the whole patient, and your response. This tool is often used not only to teach empathy but also, in part, to reduce the likelihood of malpractice claims. Bolognini and Macnaughton suggest empathy has come to imply something we "do" on behalf of the other, rather than how we "be" with our patients.

Karen Maroda (2021), in her chapter on *Myths about empathy and mirror neurons,* holds that our view of empathy has been seriously compromised and that we have lost our minds and our honest reactions and responses with our patients in our pull toward being the all caring, well-attuned therapist. She states bluntly, "the assumption that the analyst's experience of empathy routinely produces a therapeutic response is essentially false" (p. 141). And goes on to say,

In spite of research saying it is perfectly normal to react negative to another person's aggressive feelings...we somehow think we should be above 'these' normal responses. Our guilt and shame about reacting negatively to our patient's creates fertile ground for inauthentic responses.

(p. 160)

Our patients need to know we can be penetrated, put off balance, and that we can access love, hate, and the full range of human emotions and reactions that emerge within the relationship and *use* them to further growth for the patient. Macnaughton, as noted above, suggests that we need to "recomplicate" the word. I suggest that we move along from the term entirely. As I understand contemporary relational psychoanalysis with its emphasis on interpersonal conflicts, enactments, and working through, I experience a model that requires a robust deeply human authentic encounter. As two distinct subjectivities grapple to find meaning through contrast and difference, it is not the therapist's empathic efforts that matter, it is their authenticity. This is an authenticity that involves a full embodiment of the therapist's mind and their affective experiences. And when we do show up, honestly and authentically, the patient is generally relieved.

## Affect and Intuition

Intuition, our sixth sense, is that which is aroused within our viscera, our instincts, our inner voice, and our inner wisdom. Regrettably, psychotherapy has not acknowledged intuition as a primary therapeutic function. Yet, the truth is, most therapy is primarily conducted using our intuitions as our guide.

Malcom Gladwell (2006), author of the popular book *Blink: the Power of Thinking without Thinking,* discovered that spontaneous intuitive decisions are often as good as—or even better than—carefully planned and considered ones. Too much information can interfere with the accuracy of a judgment, and can in fact, corrupt good judgment. Gladwell explains that better judgments are executed by simplicity and frugality. We must value the power of what shows up intuitively and let our patient in on our intuitive experiences so we can be co-metabolizers together.

If intuition is thoughtfully employed and strategically placed in the therapeutic space for both therapist and patient to navigate, it acts as a bridge between the conscious and the unconscious. Drawing attention to our intuitive affective senses opens the pathway for exploration between the known and the unknown where our intuition serves as a conduit toward intersubjective play as we offer what we sense directly with our patients.

## Affect and the Unconscious

Dissociated affected states are lodged within the unconscious in a sub-symbolic state (without words) and show up affectively through dreams and intuitions. We may think of the unconscious as the container of cut-off affective parts of the self. In the MAMAL approach, participants are asked to pay close attention to their intuitions, to the uncanny that occurs within the therapeutic relationship, as well as the dreams of the patient and of the therapist holding to the understanding that the "unconscious of one human being react(s) upon that of another, without passing through the conscious" (Freud, 1923, p. 19). Further,

> by voluntarily and consciously taking over the psychic sufferings of the patient, [we are exposed] to the overpowering contents of the unconscious and hence also to their inductive action...The patient, by bringing an activated unconscious content to bear upon the doctor, constellates the corresponding unconscious material in him.
>
> (Jung, 1946, p. 176)

Therefore, in working with the unconscious the clinician not only observes the patient's free associations but also their own, following their intuition, is willing to be surprised, and is willing to suffer that which comes upon them, bending their own unconscious life "like a receptive organ towards the transmitting unconscious of the patient" (Freud, 1923, p. 15).

Attention is given to these unconscious affective states by surrendering to the therapist's own unconscious mental activity and by attending to gestures, tone of voice, affects, animations, nervous laughter, and the uncanny occurring within themselves and within their patient. While probing the dreams of their patients, relational psychodynamic therapists explore their own dreams that may emerge in relationship to their patient. Each of these efforts provides clues to that which is embedded deep within psychic structure where we gain access to the unconscious and disassociated aspects of the patient.

## Affect Integration vs. Affect Regulation

Affect regulation practiced in cognitive-behavioral therapies focuses on the *management* of emotion (e.g., anger management). In contrast, psychodynamic approaches seek to *reactivate* emotion, as the emotion becomes more labile, unregulated, reenacted, and open to integration. Rather than seeking to control emotions, the goal in psychodynamic therapy is to increase the capacity to process and influence the multiple affective states that ebb and flow throughout the life of a person.

While both regulation and integration play crucial roles, affect regulation is especially well-suited for addressing heightened emotional situations involving uncontrollable anger, abuse toward others, and self-harm. Models of affect regulation, such as EMDR, Mindfulness, CBT, and DBT, temporarily regulate emotions but the effectiveness of affect regulation is often short-term, especially if the intervention lacks concurrent relational experience. Ultimately, however, negative affective states need to be consciously experienced, reworked, and integrated into the individual's overall psyche for lasting impact.

Movement toward integration progresses within psychotherapy through moments of resonance and attunement as well as through disruption and restoration. It is the therapist's responsibility to address the moment-by-moment affective states, often unconscious, occurring within themselves and within the therapeutic dyad. If the therapist is willing to courageously work with the affective states that emerge within the therapeutic relationship, integration of dissociated parts of the self is brought out in the open and into the light. When this occurs, emotions are not only regulated but have also the chance to be integrated into the complex emotional life of the patient. This complexity allows for a nuanced understanding of multiple emotional states, improving the patient's capacity to reflect and hold the tension of opposing views, enhancing their resilience and tolerance for managing multiple affective states, and may even increase openness toward relationships, historical and current, which have been and are the source of their dysregulation.

### Therapist Dysregulation

A student once stated, "When I become affectively dysregulated, I freak out, and you don't seem to. Why?"

I responded that I also freak out and dysregulate! But her question did prompt me to reflect on how I find my way back into the space of intersubjective play when I have been emotionally disrupted. There were three things that came to my mind. First, I expect to be dysregulated. The only way to understand our patients is to become dysregulated. If at times I do not feel uneasy, uncertain, confused, afraid, conflicted, then I am not present and have cut off my emotional responses toward my patient. Second, I know my gig, meaning when I get dysregulated, I know that my tendency is to either retreat and go silent or to dominate the session with words, advice, counsel, and explanations. When I catch myself doing this, I know that I am acting out of my dysregulation rather than being in it and exploring it. Consequently, as I begin to explore my dysregulation, I return to the basic principle of "What the hell is going on here anyway?" and begin to ask, "What does this dysregulation have to do with the patient's story?" "How is this state related to the relational patterning of our relationship?" "How is it linked to my own story, and how can I use this experience to better understand my patient's narrative?" This basic principle of radical openness toward myself and toward my patient assists me in getting back on my feet. Lastly, my theoretical stance is that moments of dysregulation are to be brought into the therapeutic relationship and explored together and co-metabolized. With the knowledge that this dysregulation is therapeutic, and we can talk about it, anchors me.

### Therapist Burnout

Unless the therapist affectively enters into a relationship with their patient, is willing to be moved by the patient's story, and participates in the positive and negative energies flowing through the relationship, the treatment is only partly engaged, compromising the depth of what psychological treatment can provide. When therapists report to me that they are burning out and need a break, their eyes often roll when I say, "I think you need to lean in more, not less. You don't need a break from; you need a break-in."

When we feel conflicted in our work, we tend to pull back, lean on our theories, our supposed expertise, and distance ourselves from the patient and ourselves. By digging deeper into our emotional reactions, we usually discover something replicated within the patient's story. Our story and their story colliding, breaking up, but also connecting, resuscitates the treatment giving potential for deeper understanding.

When we keep avoiding and pushing away what is right in front of us—that is the potential of working with what is happening between two human beings, is exhausting. But when we keep playing and engaging our affects and our mind and have the courage to make ourselves more visible and show up more, the work becomes invigorating.

### In Summary

RPT turns the mind-body equation upside down recognizing that to have a good mind about something, affective states of being need full voice. Thus, the MAMAL method is affect-focused first, understanding that we have a feeling about something before we have a mind about it. However, we are also mindful that though we feel first, our task as therapist is to also have a mind about our affect. We keep in mind, however, that our mind often takes over too quickly, casting itself as the authority of the self, offering defensive rational solutions that often deny our affective states. Acknowledging that the mind often operates defensively as a protection against our fears, we seek to hold both mind and affect in check. Though we can appreciate the mind's protection and its role to synthesize and categorize, we must also consider that in particularly highly aroused negative affective experiences the mind's protection actively denies these affective states. Our task as therapists, as we confront defensive structures such as splitting and denial, is to assist the mind to consider the cut-offs laboring in our unconscious which are affectively experienced, knowing that when unconscious repressed self-states are revived, they can be re-imagined.

Psychotherapy's gift is to privilege the affect over the mind to strip away the layers and defenses that are impediments toward a vibrant self. And to do this, we must be alive to ourselves, our bodies, our affect, and our minds. We listen from our *viscera*, attending with our whole being and with full involvement in the relational psychodynamic process.

**PART FOUR: METABOLIZATION**

### From Affect to Mindedness

Metabolization is the place where theory meets experience.

When first exposed to the MAMAL method encouraging the use of their affect, participants describe this way of working as a profoundly liberating experience. Traditionally trained to set aside their subjectivity and to objectively analyze the emotional landscape of their patients, this new realization of using their affective experience as the primary avenue of understanding the internal and social world of their patients proves to be a transformative revelation.

After being introduced to the practice of metabolization, the process of taking raw subjective emotion, then swirling it around in one's mind, and connecting it to their affective experiences, newly trained RPT participants often become disheartened when told affect, though powerful, *isn't* everything. They report that bringing their unmetabolized subjective emotions directly to their patient, though frightening, is what has energized their work. The concern they share is that if they shift out of their affective reveries and move into thinking about their experience, the fire that has been ignited will be extinguished. While I acknowledge this concern, psychotherapy is not psychotherapy unless there is a mindedness of our affective experiences. The key is holding both affective experience and thinking simultaneously. Affect is the force that propels our minds to think. Feeling our deep affective experiences helps us to locate our patient and our mind.

And though I feel more comfortable with risking articulating unmetabolized affect than I do with highly sophisticated well-thought precise interpretations void of the therapist's subjectivity, our professional training has also prepared us to have a mind about our affects. We offer our mind to stimulate the mind of our patient into the space of intersubjective play where the analytic couple co-metabolize, searching for connections and meaning together.

Italian psychoanalyst Armando Ferrari offers us a way out of the mind/body, either/or dilemma, by suggesting the embodiment of the two – the body and the mind. He says, the body is not only the mind's first object," [affect first] "but is the object out of which mind originates" (as cited in Carignani, 2012, p. 289), meaning that the body must also be thought.

Metabolization is that in-between place of attending to the emotions that have been elicited in the therapist-patient encounter and finding our words to speak to them. In this liminal space, we ponder, catch our breath, organize, and sort. The art of metabolization is the therapist's capacity to hold on to: the multiple affective states, unconscious awakenings, and shifting relational experiences brought about within the therapeutic relationship. A good question to ask, especially in heightened affective states, is "What the hell is going on here anyway!?"

Though thoughtful and objective interpretation has been the general work-horse of psychoanalytic therapy, when working within a relational model, we reorient and discipline ourselves toward the subjective affective experiences, experienced within the therapeutic relationship and try to guard against objectifying the patient and valorizing brilliant interpretations. Our guide in assessing effective metabolization is determined by whether our articulations of our subjectivity in direct relationship to the patient's subjectivity deepens affective states and does not obliterate them. We are also able to gauge patient-therapist interactions if there is a movement toward deeper self-reflection and imagination.

## Case Formulation vs. Metabolization

It is easy to confuse case formulation with metabolization. Simply put, case formulation is primarily a *cognitive* function focusing our attention on assessment related to the patient's presenting problem. Metabolization is an *affective* function that emerges within the therapeutic pair and connects the mind and affects to help understand the patient.

In case formulation, the therapist considers the patient's presenting illness as well as the event(s) that brought them to treatment. Clinicians are trained in the use of the Mental Status Exam that considers the patient's affect, thought processes, level of consciousness, presentation of self, capacity for insight and judgement, the patient's strengths and limitations, psychosocial and medical history, substance abuse, medications, interpersonal relations, occupational history and evaluation of the patient's family of origin and any traumatic events that occurred such as sexual abuse, neglect, and violence. Culture and traditions are also now more frequently included in case formulation.

These evaluations are standard in our practices and useful, but they often lead to categories in which to diagnose the patient and triaged manualized treatment protocols in which to engage them. The problem, however, is that the human condition is not easily categorized. Deep within each human person is a fundamental desire/yearning to be seen in their own uniqueness and peculiarities. I have found that unless a behavioral intervention or a piece of advice I may offer is connected to my felt experience, unique to the patient's story, the intervention fails.

The term "metabolization" emerged in the sciences in the 1800s by physiologist Theodor Schwann to describe the physical and chemical responses that occur within our bodies that keep us alive and stay alive. Metabolization is an action that absorbs, digests, and breaks down processes to undergo a change.

In psychoanalysis, we turn to Wilfred Bion who helps us understand metabolization through his theories on projection and container/contained. Bion understood projection as something that communicates and resounds within the analyst's own viscera. According to him, analysts are tasked with absorbing, digesting, and containing their felt experiences, metabolizing them, and subsequently offering an interpretation of the patient's projections. Bion's challenge was to assimilate unmetabolized raw affective experiences (beta elements) projected "into" the therapist and transform them into symbolized thoughts manifested in the capacity for self-reflection (alpha elements). Bion's ideas were connected to the vital role of a mother's capacity to withstand the baby's projections, attune to them, contain them, think about them, and return them to the baby in a way in which the baby can tolerate their split-off emotional states. Metabolization was intended for the analyst to sort and make sense of the projections and to provide an appropriate relevant interpretation to the intrapsychic structures of the patient. Though Bion re-imagined projection as a means of communication in contrast to Freud and Melanie Klein who viewed projection as defense, his thinking remained one-dimensional. The projective communication implied only what the patient projected to the analyst. It did not consider the analyst's own subjectivity and projections as essential to the communication process.

Projection, much like the terms *transference* and *countertransference*, are so embedded in our lexicon and shared across the psychoanalytic discipline that it is not possible to erase them from our theoretical canon. Nor do we need to, as projection is a powerful affective experience that goes deep within us; it hurts, confounds, and stirs us up. But as in every good theory, theories can be rethought and broadened, as in relational psychoanalytic theory where

> Projection and projective identification [have been] gradually replaced with references to enactment, where patient and analyst join together, unconsciously, to mutually generate past conflicts that have become uniquely alive in the present.
>
> (Maroda, as cited in Barsness, 2018, p. 165)

Let's take a further look at how relational theory has expanded upon Bion's thinking.

First, Bion conceptualized projection as a channel for communication. Relational theory builds upon this idea by recognizing the bidirectional nature of these communications. In this perspective, therapists and patients engage in a dialogue, seeking to explore and expand the patient's mind and narrative through the "projected" experiences of the other.

Bion emphasized the significance of embodying the patient's experience within the therapeutic relationship, absorbing these encounters into our own beings and making meaning from them. Central to Bion's theory is the concept of container/contained where the analyst metabolizes, *in their own mind,* the projections they have received. From relational psychoanalytic theory, viewed through intersubjectivity, metabolizing involves *two minds*—the mind of the therapist and the mind of the patient. While therapists receive, feel, and metabolize the patient's projections, the therapeutic process is not merely about returning modified projections to the patient. Rather, it involves placing the emotions, thoughts, and entanglements resulting from projections and enactments into the intersubjective space to be co-metabolized. In this dynamic space, the therapist considers the possibilities of their own projections, acknowledging their role in the unfolding of the therapeutic encounter. Although therapists indeed absorb projections of the uncontainable, they digest (metabolize) them with a nuanced approach. Relational therapists acknowledge the imperfection of their digestive system, recognizing that countertransference and affective states are a blend of personal issues and those of the patient.

Finally, RPT acknowledges that therapists cannot fully contain all projections and return them to the patient in a digestible manner. As projections are seen as a means of communication, it is expected that both the patient and the therapist metabolize and talk about them together. Working in this dialogical space miscommunications, impasses, interlocks, and enactments are expected and when worked through are seen as the major catalyst for change.

## Metabolization and Linking and Patterning

### Linking to the Patient's Past

I was recently asked if all therapy is replication. I stumbled for a moment, as my first response was "no." And yet, on further reflection, it seems the answer, is an unequivocal, "yes." In Freud's (1914) article, *Remembering, Repeating and Working Through,* Freud uncovered a "truth" that most have come to accept and frankly experience in their own lives. The truth is that the mind defends against trauma, dissociates itself from the trauma, loses its memory of the trauma, but unconsciously repeats the emotional upheaval over and over within the intrapsychic and interpersonal life of a person. The repetition continues negatively until the trauma is re-experienced and re-imagined. Freud referred to this psychological phenomenon as *the repetition compulsion.* Psychoanalysis was his effort to analyze the trauma as it was repeated (transferred) within the therapeutic relationship. The intent and purpose of treatment was to gain insight and agency over the traumatized past. The trauma, he claimed, is dissociated and becomes stored within the unconscious. However, though stored in the unconscious, the memory/trauma is not inactive, actively revealing itself through our dreams and our affects, and through dysregulation within interpersonal conflicts. The memory of the wrong suffered is a source of much despair, and though it can be repressed, it cannot be forgotten. The desire to repeat is to seek resolve from the pain that was caused. When it is repeated and remembered, the past is not just the past; it is an aspect of the present and of the future. Working with that which is repeated in the here and now, revives the past and links the trauma to how it is lived out in the present and imagines how it can be reimagined for the future.

The work of metabolization in the MAMAL method understands replication as a central and vital part of the treatment process. It insists that the redemption of the traumatized past occurs through the door of memory and the reworking of the past in direct relationship within the therapeutic dyad. The supervision process deeply attends to what is being repeated, recognizing that history is not just facts. It is an ache. And the history of *one* must penetrate the life of *another*. History must not only be told, but also it must be lived. When repetition does not "hit" someone (i.e., the therapist), repetition must continue until it does. It is only when the repetition activates affective states in the other and the other stays in the game and works it through that transformation can take place.

In the MAMAL method, the group diligently pursues what is being replicated in the here and now relationship with the therapist. They do so with the understanding that in the act of repetition, the patient is seeking to make contact with the therapist to locate past traumas as well as to practice new forms of relatedness. As the supervisor and group members practice metabolizing, they turn their attention to considering the patient's development. This includes the formation within the womb, the birthing process, and the attachment to primary caregivers. They also explore the development of the self over time, influenced by self-other relationships (i.e., parents, siblings, other family members, friendships, peers), significant markers in school years, significant traumas, resiliencies and growth, romantic relationships, and the patient's unique culture and traditions. Contemporary relational models seek to include consideration of sociocultural issues, social oppression and stereotypes, indigenous cultural narratives and the role of context (Tummala-Narra, 2022). We consider these formative factors of the patient as they intersect with the therapist also formed in their own early object relations, traditions, ethnicity, gender, sexuality, body, religion, and politics (see addendum 2: Mapping the Mind).

As replication is subtle and unconscious, the group members are encouraged to listen deeply to the multiple affective stirrings within themselves elicited by the patient, and to imagine how these stirrings are useful as a lens into the patient's historical relational experiences. By attuning to their own affective experience of the patient, the therapist gets a sense or a feeling of the patient's self-experience and how the patient "sets up" the therapeutic relationship and how the patient's interaction with the therapist is linked to early (object) relations (meaning how the patient used the object of the other to form a pattern of relatedness) and how the patient was used as an object by primary persons in their lives. As therapists we wonder how we are positioned as the mother, father, the sibling, and other significant others/experiences influential to the formation of the patient's life and now revived in the therapeutic relationship. We link how the patient used their objects for self-definition, as well as their experience of being used as an object by the (m)others. In therapy, we focus our attention on how the past is repeating and replicating itself in the relationship between the therapist and the patient and the various roles the patient assigns to their therapist.

### Linking to the Therapist's Own Story

As the patient's story unfolds, the therapist's own personal story is aroused. Often referred to as countertransference, which is often ignored, or if noted, not used productively. However, the therapist's arousal of their own affective states is an essential, unavoidable, and useful aspect of psychodynamic treatment. What is aroused within the therapist almost always has something to do with the patient's story. The patient, usually unconsciously, finds their therapist through the therapist's vulnerability. So, the therapist asks, "How is this awakening of my own story linked to the patient's story?" "Why is this patient needing to pull from this part of my story?" "How can knowing my story help me show up with this patient?" Understanding the usefulness of the therapist's own subjectivity is guided by holding to the notion that the therapist's affective arousal has been occasioned by this patient at this specific time and therefore is distinctive to this patient's story. This stance does not eliminate the possibility that the arousal has little to do with the patient and is, in fact, unrelated to the patient and is a personal issue of the therapist. But even then, we are careful not to quickly dismiss the experience, because we are closest to our patient's story when we are closest to our own.

### Linking to the Emergent Patterns Within the Therapeutic Relationship

The relationship that grows between the patient and the therapist is another area of keen interest. Of course, the patterns of the past repeat; but every new relationship begins to pattern in its own distinct way. Thinking and feeling is interactional; and as the session weaves together its own distinct way of relating, we pay close attention to the emergent patterns within the therapeutic dyad. Knoblauch (2018) describes the patterns that emerge uniquely within the therapeutic relationship as a "polyrhythmic weave, likening psychoanalysis to the music of the samba, 'highlighting in the subtle micro-moments of a clinical interaction... [and how the original tune varies] inspired by changing affective states, bodily sensations and nuance (pp. 142–143). By paying attention to contradictions, gaps in the conversation, fluctuations in the body, silences, or too much talking, the therapist is getting a sense as to how they and their patient are dancing with each other. As we keep track of the session, we begin to see how we are being pulled into the patient's story. When we are "in," we are better able to participate in understanding the story and in the rewriting of it. Or in other words to dance to the music of the analytic samba.

### Linking Parallel Process

A common occurrence within the MAMAL consultation is the phenomenon of parallel processes. What parallel process simply means is that the presenter of the muse and group members begin to act and respond in a similar pattern to the case being presented. Let us say the presenter is expressing hopelessness with their case. The group may find themselves lost and hopeless and without emotion or thought, paralleling analogous emotions to that of the presenter. A rich learning experience can happen when the group can catch themselves in a parallel process and begin to imagine how they got there and what they might do about it among themselves and subsequently how they might imagine working with it with their patient.

## A Metabolizing Structure: A Mapping of the Mind

During a supervision session it is common following an articulation for someone to ask me, "Can you tell me how you got there?" Essentially asking me, "What goes on in your mind that assists you in forming your articulation?" In addition to the Metabolization Map found in the Addendum 2, I offer the following map of my own mind. My mind is mapping:

- the affective stirrings activated within me elicited from my patient and to my affective experiences, particularly those I wish to avoid.
- how the therapeutic relationship between us is patterning and how this pattern may be linked to the patient's formative years, their culture, traditions, sociocultural issues, traumas, developmental arrests, attachments, the patients' resiliencies and how these influencers have formed this patient's view of themselves and their interpersonal style of relatedness. I attempt to discern the roles assigned to me. I wonder how I might be influencing our interactions.
- the patient's early object relations, their family relations, and relations with significant others. I try to imagine what it would be like to be my patient and how others in relationship to my patient experience them.
- how the past is repeating itself in the present.
- key words and phrases that resonate and draw my attention as well the gaps, contradictions, and dissociations within the patient's narrative and within our own patterns of relating.
- the uncanny and how the unconscious shows up in unexpected places both within the patient and me. I pay attention not only to the dreams of the patient but also to my own. I pay attention to the unusual thoughts that pass through my mind, asking what do these thoughts and feelings have to do with the patient?
- how is the patient's personal narrative activating me? And wonder, why? why now? why with this patient? What has this got to do with anything? Why is my story in "here?"
- the inevitable conflicts that emerge from misreads and ruptures, and working them through as a means of understanding and growth.

Using the MAMAL method participants are encouraged to consider their own map of their mind that aims to delve into the root of the patient's suffering by identifying with it, attending to the associated emotions elicited within the therapist, consider the patient's narrative as it is being replicated and the patterns and links from the past to the present and now evident within the therapeutic relationship and enter into an authentic dialogue with the patient. It is this mindedness that encapsulates the act of metabolization.

And when we "freeze" or get lost in our work, returning to our maps (i.e., how we metabolize our affective and interpersonal interactions) will guide us in our work.

## Summary

In the MAMAL method when we are metabolizing, we often have to remind ourselves of the primacy of affect as it is easy to get stuck in our minds. When the mind takes over Bryan Nixon (2019, personal communication) reminds us that,

> we must continually cultivate a capacity to tolerate experience without too quickly collapsing into formulation or interpretation of meaning. When we catch ourselves offering advice or naming something for the patient, we would do well to reflect on what we may be attempting to soothe within ourselves. In that discomfort within ourselves there are clues to what may be unconsciously repeating itself between the therapist and the patient. Foreclosure of meaning is often a defensive maneuver on the part of the therapist.

It is safer to think. To *do* rather than *be*. As we move on to the next chapter where we look at the practice of articulating to our patients our metabolized affective experiences, we are forewarned that it is easier to interpret than it is to engage in "dramatic dialogues" (Atlas & Aron, 2018). Though thoughtful and objective, interpretation has been at the core of psychoanalytic practices. However, when working the relational model within a MAMAL consultation we constantly seek to reorient and discipline ourselves toward the subjective, affective experiences occurring within the therapeutic relationship aligned with the words that we bring to our patients. We do so to guard against objectifying the patient and overvaluing our brilliant interpretations. Our guide in assessing effective metabolization is determined by answering the question, "Has the work deepened and is the patient's capacity for self-reflection and imagination increased?"

## PART FIVE: ARTICULATION

In Chapter 1 of this text, I spoke to the genesis of the MAMAL method. I stated that when I began to ask my supervisees, "What is going on in your 'gut' when you are sitting with your patient?" I discovered a remarkable contrast between what the supervisee was doing and saying in treatment (i.e., common stuff like empathic listening, offering insights/interpretation and advice) and what they were feeling and experiencing and not saying. Sitting in their "gut" languishing were deep emotion, unworked intuitions, unconscious urgings, and relational tensions. In not speaking these felt experiences to the patient, critical psychic energy was being cut-off from the therapeutic couple. When we began to deal with the affective aspects of the clinician's experience, we found them relevant to the patient's story. When the therapist began to risk speaking more directly to the experience of the patient/therapist relationship, the treatment was enlivened. When they chose not to speak, it was detrimental not only to the patient but also to the well-being of the clinician.

Historically the subjectivity of the therapist was left out of the clinical space. However, within RPT, it is acknowledged that it is not only impossible to park one's subjectivity at the door but also that in doing so a wealth of clinical data is lost.

Consequently, by attending to the therapist's own subjectivity, the patient's subjectivity, and the dynamics of the in-between (intersubjectivity), navigating therapeutic space becomes quite complex. Particularly, questions arise such as how much of the self of the therapist is to be disclosed, and how does their therapeutic mind differ from the patient's mind? Some critics fear that working intersubjectively is a somewhat undisciplined process where therapist's random self-disclosures and excessive emoting of the therapist's personal affective states dominates the treatment. There also exists a misconception that the therapist and patient are primarily engaged in working out their relational issues in much the same way they might with friends or other social relations. A question sometimes asked is, "Whose analysis is this anyway?"

It is true that a relational process without a structure could be misconstrued. However, the discipline of the therapist attending to their own subjective experience in relation to their patient and through the act of authentic expression provides a structure that exceeds any social relation, transforming the therapeutic relationship into a unique and profound connection.

From a relational psychodynamic perspective, human growth is predicated on the fact that we need the mind and genuine experience of another to grow. We need a similar subject, who is also distinct and separate, in order to find ourselves. As we deconstruct the mind of the therapist, in contrast to the mind of the patient (who is only required to bring their story as they know and experience it), there is one basic "rule" required of the therapist. The rule being that the therapist must consider all that passes through them as informational value in relationship to their patient.

We come to understand our patients by turning "our unconscious like a receptive organ toward the transmitting unconscious of the patient..." (Freud, 1923, p. 15). As the patient speaks, we take "notes" on our experiences, attend to our intuitions, notice what is being aroused in our own story, and track the pulls and pressures that are evoked as we trace the patterns and links that are evoked within both our unconscious and our conscious minds. We turn our reveries toward the patient's narrative as it is being told and is unfolding within the therapeutic relationship.

Linked to these "notes" is the art and practice of articulation. By having access to the therapist's unique mind spoken on their behalf, the patient is given a glimpse into how their intrapsychic and interpersonal world is experienced and perceived by a contrasting other. As the therapist offers access to their mind and experience, the patient is also invited to be curious about the therapist's mind and to express their experience of the therapist. Much is revealed of the patient's story when they are able to speak about their experience of the therapist. This is a vital component of the therapeutic experience. It is the examination of these two minds (intersubjectivity) in the reciprocal process of inquiry which leads toward growth and change. RPT understands that our patients know themselves best, they just don't know that they know, and they seek us out to help them discover what they already know. Bollas (1987) says it this way:

> There is in each of us a fundamental split between what we think we know and what we know but may never be able to think. In the course of transference and countertransference the psychoanalyst may be able to facilitate the transfer of the unthought known into thought, and the patient will come to put into thought something about his being which he had not been able to think up until then
>
> (p. 282)

Thus, it is our job to explore with our patients what they cannot trust in their own mind and to help them know what they know but are fearful of knowing. This is made possible by offering our patients a level of honesty about what's going on in our minds and our affects in relationship to them, as it evolves within the therapeutic process.

The relational psychodynamic therapist holds to the notion that a patient needs to hear what is on the therapist's mind and how the therapist experiences them. Brad Strawn and I refer to this as Courageous Speech/Disciplined Spontaneity (2018) where the therapist is encouraged to take risks by stating what has come to their mind within the context of the therapeutic relationship. Risky though their speech may be, the therapist offers their ideas from a non-authoritarian stance with tentativeness, curiosity, and humility. Words are offered to the patient with a spirit of inquiry, exploration, and negotiation. As most methods are cautious in articulating to the patient their experience of the patient, this is one of the most difficult shifts to make when working within a relational model.

Articulation in MAMAL consultation groups takes risks of articulating the therapist's subjective experience by practicing speaking their experiences out loud. Neil Altman explores the act of articulating in this way:

> ...though I am not sure-footed, there is only one way to find out about his (speaking of a patient) coherence and his ability to link and that is by bringing my experience to him. I am reminded of Ogden's chapter on the initial interview in his text, *The Primitive Edge of Experience*. He says, people say to be cautious what we say, because we don't know what the patient can tolerate. Ogden differs on this however, and believes that the question in the patient's mind is, "how much can you tolerate?" It seems important to go for the deepest level from the get-go. What the patient is trying on or what is really going on in the patient's mind is "is there a place here for me?" Anna Freud said we must calibrate how much of the patient's anxiety we expose. I would say if you have to do that, you are more likely calibrating how much anxiety you want to be exposed to. I had a supervisor once say to me, you can say anything you like if you know why you said it. This does not work however, because we do not know why things come to our mind, or why we say them. We do not know where these thoughts come from. We may have no idea. So, we put it out there. The reason we put it out there is because we are trying to get a 'scent' and 'inkling' of where this is coming from.
>
> (Barsness, 2018, p. 179)

The primary practice of articulation in the supervision model aims to broaden the articulator's experience of the patient and to further metabolize and experience deeper affective states in response to the patient. The purpose is not to rehearse what a therapist might say to the patient. Practicing articulating in this way grows each group members' confidence in speaking more courageously and authentically. Their fear of speaking authentically diminishes when they recognize that the relational model is predisposed to working collaboratively where our words are used for further inquiry rather than as truth. The therapist's interventions, interpretations, and thoughts come as conversations and are inherently unpredictable and unformulated.

Seasoned relational psychoanalysts who participated in a qualitative research study on psychoanalytic technique (Barsness, 2018) spoke of articulation in this way:

> Sometimes things just fly out of my mouth, which if I am there to explore this with the patient and it is connected to our experience, it is what is needed; How do we know anything? By talking about what has happened; I know that I can't have clarity unless I say something; I recognize that because I am working with experience, the timing is always right because I am stating what it is that is happening; I think that in

some form the patient already knows what I am thinking anyway; I do a lot of reflecting out loud. I suppose I am modeling the idea of looking inside while speaking outside.

(p. 181)

When to speak and how to say what we experience remains challenging, but it is evident that the relational analyst chooses to let the patient in on their thoughts believing that in doing so the work is advanced. It is upon this foundation that MAMAL consult groups direct their attention away from interpretation and into complex dialogue.

I vividly recall a supervisory session led by a highly esteemed analyst gifted in language and insight in which I was a participant. While moved and envious of the interpretations he offered, I was also struck by his lack of affect and this absence troubled me. I realized I could not sense the supervisor's emotions which I imagined had informed his well-thought-out interpretation. Despite being captivated by his brilliant mind, I felt disturbed by his detachment from his own feelings.

While the function of the mind is to sort and make sense of our emotions, the emotion that stimulated the mind often gets left behind or discounted in the process. This is especially true in heightened affective moments of eroticism and aggression where the mind takes over by dissociating disruptive feelings through intellectualization. Winnicott (1971) warned against intellectualization when he stated, "that interpretation outside the ripeness of the material is indoctrination and produces compliance" (p. 51). He believed that resistance arises [when] interpretation is given outside the overlap of the patient's and analyst's playing together. Winnicott's idea of play emerged from his work with children, and the actions that "constitute love between two imperfect people" (Nussman, 2012, p. 282). Winnicott felt that our thoughts were meant to be played with and not considered as official versions of the truth. Bollas (1987) suggests we put our thoughts:

to the patient in such a way that he does not feel himself to be cornered... and believe that it can be valuable for the clinician to report selected subjective states to his patient for mutual observation and analysis... so long as the analyst does so in the overall interest of the analysis and s/he tunes into and offers further thoughts about the patient's response to such "disclosure." The act of shifting our interpretations is *not* about transgressing professional boundaries; it *is* about being prepared to share the grounds of one's own thinking with the person you are thinking about.

(p. 206)

Detachment from our emotions leads to formulaic explanations where the transformative energy becomes diluted in carefully crafted words. Consequently, the connections to the patient's narrative and the unfolding live

narrative of the patient/therapist dyad is lost. In the MAMAL process, we practice speaking aloud what is on our minds about our patient to grow our ability
to speak from our felt experience. What assists group members in growing the
courage to speak from their "heart" more honestly is to remind them that we
hold to a stance that our words are an invitation to play.

By attending to our bodies, to what we are feeling, observing facial expressions, body movements, inflections, and tone of voice, we get a good read of
our patient. Yet it remains an imperfect one. And "it is an 'open' secret that
patients look 'into the soul' of the analyst" (Jung, 1913, p. 198) and that they
are also 'read[ing] the analyst's character intuitively' (1914, p. 260). But the
patient's read is also an approximation. It is in the deconstructing of these two
reads (the analyst's and the patient's) that is at the center of the therapeutic
process. It is in the working through of our misreads where most psychotherapy takes place. Arthur Feiner in his article Reads and Misreads (1988) says:

> In the end the patient uses the analyst's failures, often quite small ones,
> perhaps maneuvered by the patient and we have to put up with being
> misunderstood even hated...it is the failure ...that is singled out as im-
> portant on account of its being a reproduction of the original and [it is
> the failure and through the repair] that will create new growth.
>
> (p. 645)

Knowing our words are an approximation and are often a misread, we invite
the patient into a dialogue with the intent of mutual exploration. The goal is
to grow confidence in our therapeutic conversations:

> enough to act on impulse and mistrust ourselves enough to pause and
> reflect. Technique, has to do with self-reflection, reflection in action,
> reflection before action and reflection after action, balancing the her-
> meneutics of suspicion with the hermeneutics of faith with an emphasis
> on mutuality, mutual influence, mutual recognition, mutual accommo-
> dation, mutual negotiation and mutual change, which of course implies
> the uniqueness of each person and each dyad and our community of
> other selves and dyads.
>
> (Lew Aron, 1998, p. 119)

Therapists consider their thoughts and affects and attempt to metabolize before they speak and while they are speaking. They are also willing to make a
mistake in speaking given their predisposition to understanding therapy as a
conversation rather than mere analytic interpretation and to present oneself
to the other "free of the desire for semblance [image], there is brought into
being a memorable common fruitfulness which is to be found nowhere else"
(Buber, in Agassi, 1999, p. 76).

To speak courageously, we need a healthy respect for anxiety and tension without feeling threatened. We hold direct requests for acknowledgment

non-defensively and with curiosity. We value our words as a means for exploration rather than as correctness. We hold firmly but lightly and follow the flow of the analyst-patient relationship recognizing that what we *say* to our patients is second in command to how we *work* with what is said and experienced in the interplay of the dyad. We play, we wonder, and we ask, "Has collaborative inquiry increased and is our patient freer to engage more deeply with themselves and with others?"

Though at times our words may be hurtful, it is often just as true that what we do not say may cause harm. When the patient and the therapist understand together that our words are considered as words for inquiry, a sense of safety is established promoting a deeper analysis of the patient's internal and interpersonal world. When patients experience us as persons willing to risk our experience of them, they are emotionally moved, not offended.

There will be times when the patient does not respond favorably to our articulation, or we have misspoken. In these moments, it is common for the therapist to jump to repair the suspected damage. While an apology might be warranted, a too quick apology is generally in the service of the therapist's anxiety and guilt. We should first consider that the words we spoke may have value when reflected upon with the patient. So, we must be cautious not to quickly collapse into assuming we erred and start soothing the patient, which most often is an attempt to soothe ourselves. We must keep in mind that the articulation that emerged, emerged from within the therapist's experience of the patient. And though it may be disruptive, it holds potential for transformation through the efforts of the therapeutic couple working through the disruption caused by the words.

Within the context of supervision/consultation, the act of articulation may give the impression that we are always looking for the right words to say to the patient. Articulation in the MAMAL method, however, is not so much about finding the right words, but to further expand our minds and affective experiences about ourselves and our patients. By hearing ourselves speak, a deeper sense of what we are feeling emerges and a greater connection to what our patients may be experiencing is achieved. Supervisors often must remind themselves and the group members that the practice of articulation has nothing at all to do with finding the right words! Rather, we practice articulation to listen to ourselves "out loud" where our words may shock us or further clarify for us our emotions and lead us into a deeper reflection on the therapeutic process.

## Self-Disclosure

### Introduction

In the chapter entitled: *Courageous Speech/Disciplined Spontaneity* in the text, *Core Competencies in Relational Psychoanalysis* (Barsness & Strawn, 2018) we say that "all therapy is disclosure" (p. 182), considering that we are always disclosing either consciously or unconsciously what is on our mind, how our mind works, what affective states are present and how it relates to the patient. In the back and forth of conscious and unconscious experiences, we encourage that the analyst strives to speak courageously, bearing an authentic witness to the unfolding events occurring within the therapeutic relationship (pp. 182–183). Everything we do is a form of self-disclosure, so it seems wise to talk about it rather than try to convince ourselves that we can hide it. As the therapist's experience is linked to the patient in both subjective and inter-subjective ways, we quote Bromberg who believes that "unconscious affects, thoughts and fantasies are dissociated in both patient and therapist so they must be processed through conversation in order to bring them into 'cognitive symbolization through language.' Transference-countertransference enactment is the process by which patients dissociated self-states, or what Bromberg calls 'trauma-derived emotion schemas' make themselves known" (p. 182). Consequently, because conscious and unconscious affects, thoughts, and fantasies are co-created in the analytic dyad, the therapist must put their own experience into words for the patient to make sense of what they have dissociated. Bromberg states:

> The patient's pressure to force the analyst to give up his right to privacy is organized not simply by a need to know the analyst, but by a wish to know what the analyst knows about the patient but has dissociated.
>
> (p. 183)

This creates a situation that Owen Renik (in Barsness & Strawn, 2018, p. 183), refers to as *flying blind*. Flying blind is admitting that all we really know is our experience of being with the patient, and subsequently we do not know with certainty what will provide a corrective experience. If patients' perceptions/feedback are ignored or interpreted away, or if patients are forced to explore without the therapist's authentic response, dialogue is effectively shut down and the dissociated will stay inaccessible. Furthermore, therapists must place their perceptions of themselves, the client, and their interaction on the table, which may require the "analyst to say a good deal about him or herself – sometimes more than is comfortable" (Barsness & Strawn, 2018, p. 183). When the analyst plays their cards "face up," it invites an opportunity for the analytic dyad to compare, contrast, and explore their perceptions. Karen Maroda (in Barsness & Strawn, 2018) suggests, "the only tenable position for us to adopt is to focus on the nature of the interaction and the emotional states of the therapist and the patient…" (p. 183) and for the therapist and patient to talk about it.

The patient is mostly interested in my experience of them and acknowledging our experience, together, not my personal self-disclosures. In the case studies that Brad and I presented in the chapter—both cases referring to erotic tension—we realized that the disclosures that we made and compelled to share, were in the end not necessarily personal self-disclosures, but better defined as *acknowledgment*. The impasses in both cases lifted when we ac-knowledged our participation in the interlock. We learned that our patients were not interested in any personal sexual disclosure but that the erotic en-ergy we were blocking was in pursuit of making contact not in consumma-tion. Of course, erotic, and angry tensions that occur in therapy are the most worrisome. We learned that if "aspects of the analyst's unconscious partici-pation in the therapeutic drama remained unexpressed and therefore, un-explored, whole areas of the patient's unconscious experience may be kept out of full participation in the interpersonal arena of reconfigured meanings" (Dimen, 2003, p. 11).

Relational Psychoanalysis's emphasis on working directly within the af-fective energies between the therapist and the patient and talking about it, alters our understanding of self-disclosure. Relational psychoanalysis' focus on therapist's presence, affective attunement, and willingness to engage au-thentically with the patient, is better understood as disclosing the relational interactions of the therapeutic relationship. By highlighting the mutual ex-ploration of affective energies and the therapist's openness to being present in the therapeutic encounter, the self is always disclosing, but disclosing in direct relation to the interactions between themselves and their patients. Con-sequently, I have chosen to speak more regularly of *relational disclosure* to best describe our therapeutic conversations. Relational disclosure is defined as disclosing my ongoing relational experience to the patient and the impact they are having on me—and inviting them to do the same.

That said, I will address three areas of disclosure and demonstrate how each of them can be resituated and rethought into relational disclosure. The three areas I will address are: responsive self-disclosure; therapist initiated self-disclosure and disclosure of the therapist's personal life from outside sources. Within these three areas the therapist must keep in mind the vari-ous reactions patients may have. These reactions can range from increased trust and relatability to discomfort, distrust, and a shift in boundary confu-sion where the patient feels compelled to take care of the therapist or in their discomfort, leave the treatment. By attending to these reactions relationally—that is, to the interaction rather than the disclosure themselves, the therapeu-tic experience can grow.

### Area One: Responsive Self-Disclosure

When patients ask me a direct question about my own life, I have grown comfortable answering the question directly and then exploring why they wished or needed to know. Earlier in my career, I tended to do that in reverse. I think either way works. I agree with Karen Maroda, who says, "I prefer to tell patients the truth. If [they] are asking the question, [they] unconsciously already know the answer" (Maroda, 2004, p. 170). Rarely has a patient asked me a question that I felt unable to answer directly. Discussing these ques-tions together has tended to build a tenderness toward each other. I believe that, in general, patients' questions about me are an effort to make contact and that they are more interested in what is going on within our relationship (relational disclosure) rather than the specifics of my personal life (personal self-disclosure).

However, there are questions patients ask that disrupt us and confound us and whose questions are not necessarily questions seeking contact but are as a defense and a refusal to work out the fantasies they may have connected to the traumas of their past. Psychoanalyst Orna Guralnik in an interview in the New Yorker (2022) says, "she tends to keep her own romantic life private, and there's a reason behind her choice "There's so much that people gain from being able to not know about me, or from being able to imagine me as one way or another," she told *The New Yorker*. Am I a conservative straight person? Am I gay? Am I queer? The moment I start talking about myself, I'm robbing them of all that."

And from my own experience, I recall a very anxious patient who refused to look at me, turning her chair away from me and peppering me with personal questions. In that case, I suggested to her that while I might answer those questions someday, my experience of her questions was that they were a way to avoid me rather than to get to know me and a means to avoid what was deeply troubling her. I did not know how those questions would evolve over time, but I did not see engaging in a volley of questions and answers as helpful in the moment and told her so. I suggested to her that I believed something deeper was happening and until we could locate what that may be, I would hold my answers to her questions carefully. We later learned that her questions were her defense against having to talk about the severe childhood sexual abuse she suffered as well as a means of escaping her sexual feelings that were beginning to come alive in her life, including in her work with me. As the treatment progressed, her questions subsided, and those that did not, I felt comfortable answering.

In another case, a patient was curious about personal aspects of my marriage, my family, and my sexual life. He threatened to leave treatment if I did not answer these specific questions. I explained that in answering those questions, I would not only be speaking for myself but also for the intimate others in my life, and that I chose not to answer them, especially perhaps to the extent that he would like. I also said that given the intensity and threat of such questions, I was not sure I could trust him with my personal life. I emphasized that I would not answer them until we had worked through the underlying threats and said, "I do not know what disclosure might look like down the road, but for now, I am not able to directly answer your question." He left the treatment, and we never discovered the drive behind his questions. Though it could be argued that my disclosure may have helped him remain in treatment, at the time, I needed to experience a stronger bond between us before divulging deeply personal aspects of myself. I felt that our first step in working together was to work through the threat and build a sense of trust between us. I remained true to a relational position therapeutically by letting him know why I was not ready to answer his demands and that over time we could see how the questions would evolve within our work together. This is another example of relational disclosure—working with the emotional action between the two of us, in contrast to personal disclosure.

Reflecting upon the pursuit of my personal story in both these cases, I tried to not negate their quest while at the same time addressing what was happening relationally between us. In the first case by doing so, we were able to navigate ourselves closer to the patient's fears and defenses, she was able to turn her chair and face me and experience relief and enjoyment of her desires. With the second case, we were not able to get that far, but by prioritizing disclosing the relational concerns of what was happening between us, I believed directed our conversations toward, at the least, the potential good of exploring the patient's fears and aggression. As I said, I may be wrong, as the patient terminated, but it felt that the aggression within our relationship was what was driving the treatment, and no number of self-disclosures would have satisfied.

### Area Two: Therapist Initiated Self-Disclosure

I have rarely found my use of personal self-disclosure beneficial to the patient. For example, in a recent therapy session, a patient was expressing his despair about living in a beautiful but deadening "boring" city. His longing to move to a more stimulating and intellectually challenging place is currently blocked due to personal circumstances. He is at his wits' end. He also reports that no one within his community understands his dilemma or even cares. This resonated with my own past story. In my attempt to assure him I understood, I said, "I know," and proceeded to tell him about my eagerness to flee my own small and narrow background and move to the city. His response was, "You do not get it! I do not need your reassurance. I need out!" And then I got it. My experience was not his. Furthermore, I have moved on, which further can frustrate our patients, as our personal self-disclosures tend to be an issue we have resolved and where we have met with success.

So, though my story had reignited by his story, its usefulness was not in my self-disclosure. A better use of the reminder of my past was to sink down into it, remember what it felt like, and allow myself to approximate what his feelings of aloneness, separateness, and despair might be. It would seem best for me to use my affective state to feel with my patient, rather than assume that my experience was the same as his.

But when I teach my stance on relational disclosure in contrast to personal self-disclosures, it is common to receive pushback as therapists report how useful they have found self-disclosures to be in their work. Following a recent presentation, a psychologist mentioned to me that he frequently discloses personal aspects of himself to his patients, perceiving self-disclosures as a "technique and as a positive intervention." When I push back, I discover the enthusiasm of self-disclosure quickly wanes when I ask about disclosure of their negative affective or erotic arousals! Maybe, his use of self-disclosure as technique works. But I am skeptical. But in fairness and faithfulness to discourse, the only way I can imagine for us to evaluate our contrasting views is for he and I both to ask, "for whose benefit was this disclosure offered, for myself or for the patient?" Reminded that "however much it might relieve the analyst to describe his state of mind to a patient, such an action should never be undertaken solely for the purpose of the analysts' self cure" (Bollas, 1987 p. 211).

That said, I submit there are situations in which an initiated therapist-self-disclosure does connect the patient and therapist effectively. For example, a patient who was grieving the loss of her parents told her therapist, a supervisee of mine, that the only thing that was holding her together was poetry. At that moment the therapist had a memory of her own when she too had experienced deep grief and shared the following, "I too love poetry, and what is coming to my mind is a memory in my own past when I was suffering, and I began to collect different pieces of poetry. Then one day, I decided to paste each of these pieces onto a door in my bedroom. That door, I remember, was not on its hinges for some reason and was set to the side of the room. I would then lay upon my bed and look at these words, and I would find comfort."

The patient exclaimed, "That is exactly how I feel!" Though this resonant response would indicate the self-disclosure went well (and I think it did), I challenged the therapist to see if the disclosure could offer more and signaled a concern that the self-disclosure seemed valorized as a good intervention and analytic inquiry about the disclosure went no further.

I first suggested that she and her patient could explore what the patient experienced in having such an intimate shared experience with the therapist. Did her experience elicit with the therapist further her feelings of grief? Of love? Trust? Distrust? Did this experience further the patient's relational life in direct relationship to the therapist?

I also suggested that self-disclosure could be used in much the same way we free associate and work with dreams. By way of example, I offered my own musings of the unhinged door. I noted that the door is unhinged, much like the patient feels unhinged, but the door is also open and filled with comforting poetry, serving as a transitional object where the patient may once again walk into a new version of her grief.

This brief musing is simply to encourage the therapist to consider furthering the development of a self-disclosure by exploring with the patient how they experienced the disclosure relationally, and to consider the self-disclosures much like we do with dreams. A self-disclosure need not stand on its own merit, rather, personal disclosures are subject to the same theoretical and clinical disciplines of exploring affective states, the unconscious, replications, and experiencing a genuine responsiveness to the patient's story.

If therapist initiated self-disclosure is practiced it seems to me the question that must be asked following a disclosure is: did the self-disclosure make contact with the patient, further the patient's own mind about themselves, and did the therapeutic relationship deepen?" Essential to personal self-disclosure, is if the disclosure is connected to the patient's story and involves the patient in understanding how the disclosure was or was not helpful. The therapist should be mindful of the reasons behind their desire to disclose and possess a personal understanding of why they believe it may be beneficial. It is also important to not overly valorize self-disclosure as an intervention, but rather to comprehend how the disclosure is linked to the patient's narrative.

### Area Three: Disclosure of the Therapist's Personal Life Through Outside Sources

Throughout the course of treatment, life events such as marriages, pregnancies, births, illnesses, deaths, and public recognitions become public and create curiosity within our patients. Therapists, their partners, or family members may also face ethical or legal complaints, provoking questions about us. Therapist's choices to be on social media platforms and the information they place into these forums is another aspect of the therapist's personal life made known. Therapists should educate themselves on the implications of their digital footprint and its impact on their practices. How we manage these life occurrences can either build or undermine trust. These inadvertent disclosures of a therapist's personal life through outside sources can complicate the therapeutic relationship. It is essential for therapists to navigate these situations with honesty, professionalism and maintain a focus on the patient's well-being.

When ethical complaints or legal issues of the therapist surface in the treatment, the best policy is to talk directly about the complaint with the patient. For example, a colleague of mine had a personal lawsuit against him years ago, where no ethical complaints or concerns were raised. The lawsuit was made public and continues to be a source of concern in his work to this day. He reports that it is still common for his patients—both initially when setting up an appointment and if they learn of the lawsuit during treatment—to ask him about it and express their concerns about these ethical and clinical issues. He is always forthright about his situation, sharing the story from his own perspective without overexplaining the "sides" inherent in a lawsuit. In situations where such information is public, it is in the best interest of the patient and the advancement of therapy to be fully transparent. My colleague has found that this approach deepens trust and advances the therapeutic process.

Most patients acquire some personal news (gossip) about their therapists and don't always know what to do with it or whether to bring it to the therapist's attention. I recall receiving "news" about my own analyst. I learned that her first husband had died, she was going through a divorce, and she was planning to remarry soon. I found this information cumbersome to hold, curious about how she navigated her private life and how it might affect our work. However, I was also leery of letting her know that I knew these things about her, so I did not. As I write this, I realize that not bringing my concerns to her fed into my own need to "bear other people's burdens," "not be intrusive," and "be kind." I believe my work with her progressed, but as I reflect now, I wish I had spoken to her about what I knew, as I see that a part of me still holds on to these feelings in my personal relations. I feel a bit sad about how much of my life has been spent taking care of others at the cost of not taking care of myself. I wonder now if working through my (grandiose) need to take care of her might have broken this strong introject in my life. Not bringing my concerns to her was my responsibility, not hers. Furthermore, she was quite open, and I believe she would have collaborated very well with me with my questions. But without my disclosure of my concerns, I hampered her in her work with me. So, this reminds me from time to time that I have a public life (as do you) that our patients know about and hold. We need to be sensitive to these public stories about ourselves and wonder at times if in some way it is in the room but not talked about and we may have to be the one to ask the patient.

## The Fear to Disclose

In a recent consult, the patient being presented was reported as having been in a ten-year marriage with a woman who reportedly disparages him, threatens to leave him, and criticizes him for being impotent. Over the years he has progressively become increasingly withdrawn, but through the efforts of therapy and exhaustion has recently begun to assert himself and reports that he now intends to leave her. He has been in therapy at the same clinic for the past few years; but as therapists rotate out, he is reassigned to incoming therapists. He has been with the current therapist for one and a half years, but she will be leaving the clinic within the next six months. At the time of this writing, he is not yet aware of her leaving. Recently, he confessed to her that he is attracted to her and has developed feelings for her.

In the MAMAL method of supervision, following the presentation of the case, each member of the consult group is asked, "As you listened to this patient's story, what emotions were stirred in you?" During the group discussion, each member expressed negative reactions toward the patient, finding him passive and his feelings of attraction unwanted. One member described his feelings as ugly. They admitted feeling judgmental of him, angry at his passivity, and deeming his erotic feelings inappropriate. I encouraged each of them to reflect on these negative emotions, considering that they might be connected to their own countertransference issues and yet related to the patient's narrative. Through this process, we began to understand how our own emotional responses mirror, to some extent, the experiences of our patients.

One participant, upon reflecting on her negative feelings toward the patient, tearfully admitted, "I feel judgmental of his passivity, just as I am judgmental of my own passivity in my relationships, and how sick I am of it." As we delved deeper into her emotions, we started to see parallels between the patient's experiences and her own. We recognized that his passivity in the face of mistreatment and rejection from therapists mirrored the struggles with assertiveness and self-advocacy in the therapist's own story.

As we addressed the discomfort surrounding the patient's feelings of attraction to his therapist, defensive comments such as "it is inappropriate," "you don't know me, how could you have these feelings," and "you can't have those feelings here" were expressed. When these reactions were examined, the group members were able to begin to realize that these feelings stemmed from their discomfort with erotic transference experiences within the therapeutic relationship. Through the process of introspection and a radical openness to the therapist's use of their self-experience, we began to contemplate the possibility of the erotic not only as a sexual advance but also as a life force.

Group members began to appreciate the deeper dynamics at play as they reflected upon their negative countertransference reactions. They started to envision how the patient's expressed attraction was linked to his pursuit of self-efficacy. This insight underscored the importance of openly attending to their affective and countertransference states in comprehending the intrapsychic and interpersonal realm of the patient. Countertransference reactions reported by the participants evolved from considering their countertransference reactions as a defensive posture to an openness toward a more courageous inquiry.

While the outcome of this case remains uncertain, there was a movement toward finding a way to participate and communicate with the patient the emotional energy present within the relationship. Should the therapist find herself unable to, she runs the risk of the patient shutting down once again and accommodating to what the patient feels his therapist is able to bear. A clear repetition of his relationship with his wife—which is also a replication of his historical narrative. We refer to this as pathological accommodation (Brandchaft, 1998), where the patient adjusts to their therapist's views and feelings to preserve the attachment felt toward their therapist. They do so at their own peril offering up their own feelings and experiences to maintain the therapist's well-being and remain in the therapist's good graces.

## Ethical Dilemma of Non-Disclosure

This case underscores the danger and the ethical quandary of relational non-disclosure. When therapists withhold the unfolding relational dynamics within the therapeutic dyad, often under the guise of containing the patient's projections, they risk overlooking the potential hazards of such actions. Non-disclosure is a handy "technique analysts' use to hide, rather than provide a therapeutic field of action" (Cole, 2006, p. 39). When a therapist internalizes a patient's projections without engaging dialogically in strongly held feelings, the projection becomes embodied and the therapist sick. The problem with avoiding disclosure and collaborative exploration of these projections, as illustrated in the case above, is that these negative reactions gradually seep into the therapy session, festering and become expressed either aggressively or dismissively.

While the literature on the ethical dilemma of non-disclosure is limited (or even non-existent), a fundamental relational psychoanalytic principle urging clinicians to confront and engage directly the affective states evoked in the interspace between the therapist and the patient keeps us on our toes. Viewing the therapeutic relationship as an intersubjective experience places primary emphasis on exploring the ongoing interaction between therapist and patient. Rather than solely interpreting defensive structures such as projection and transference phenomena as a condition of the patient, the relational approach encourages dialogue and exploration tackling the dilemma of non-disclosure directly. Within a relational model and from a shared perspective of embodiment (Anderson, 1979; Brown & Strawn, 2014) the therapeutic relationship is viewed as co-constructed and therapists are not only objects of a patient's projection but also must "recognize that the analysand and analyst variably co-create the transferential experience [and the] analyst [must be] alert to address, and acknowledge his contribution" (Fosshage, 2000, p. 34).

### Therapists' Privacy

Lastly, it is important for therapists to remember that the ethics of confidentiality apply only to the therapist, not the patient. We should only disclose personal information to our patients that we feel comfortable having known publicly. Though this may sound self-protective—and it is, which is good self-care—it is equally important that we do not place upon our patients an expectation that they are beholden to keep our story confidential. Our patients bear no responsibility for keeping what happens in our office private.

### Articulation in Supervision vs. Therapy

Perhaps this is a good time to point out the difference between practicing articulation in supervision and how we speak with our patients. A possible misunderstanding when practicing articulation during supervision is the misconception that therapy is one active volley of words executed between the patient and the therapist, that we speak without metabolizing, and that therapy is always and only about the words we speak. However, there are many moments in therapy when we experience a deep connection where there are no words, or silences are needed to gather our thoughts, a practice not usually a part of supervision. It is important to remind ourselves that in the act of psychotherapy, lying fallow, honoring silence, and discovering connection without words is an essential aspect of the treatment.

In traditional supervision, therapists are often afraid to present cases for fear of what others may think. Presentations are often forced, carefully formulated, and presented; and supervisors are often cautious and overly careful in their feedback. In the MAMAL method, participants are encouraged to experiment, to bring out loud what is on their mind, and where their words are coming from. In supervision in the MAMAL method, we practice words to deepen our affective experience, further metabolize those affective states, and increase our fluency in speaking from a relational voice. In supervision, we are intentionally undisciplined in our words, allowing us to try them out, test them, and surprise ourselves. From that vantage point we can more actively practice and learn and grow our efforts in metabolization and articulation. In encouraging the supervisor and the participants to take risks during the supervision period, we expand our feelings and thoughts about our patients in ways that perhaps have not been available to us. This urging of participants to experiment allows them to present more honestly and freely and encourages each other to similarly take risks—risks that grow their clinical mind.

When we are with our patients, we wrestle differently as we practice speaking boldly coupled with disciplined spontaneity. Though we seek to allow the patient into the mysteries of our own mind as it relates to their story, we must also remember that we "may too quickly, [in our efforts to dislodge our emotions] foreclose the necessity of unknowing that [is also] vital to analytic exchange" (Corbett, 2011, p. 640). Corbett reminds us as relational psychoanalytic clinicians of the importance of retaining other analytic practices within the realm of the spontaneous interactive nature of a relational psychodynamic practice such as:

> Containing, waiting, associating, soliciting the patient's associations, wandering into reverie, wandering back out, dreaming, debating, practicing what one might say, silently interpreting, consciously contemplating, bridging, linking, cataloging, pacing, being lost, tolerating being lost, sequencing, listening, listening through hovering attention, listening more acutely, listening with an ear of theory, inquiring, momentarily stepping out of the bond, taking a break, remaining silent, debating silence, debating theory, considering when and/or if to bring a feeling or a thought forward, and at what point in the hour, what point in the week.
> (p. 640)

### From Interpretation to Complex Dialogue

Over my thirty-five years of being a professor supervising countless practicums, case conferences, and individual supervision within my own clinical practice, I have had the opportunity to have a window into hundreds of therapists' minds and practices. The most common language spoken among psychotherapists is the language of "You." Common therapist language involves the therapist telling the patient something about what the therapist believes the patient is doing, or transference interpretations linking and telling the patient what they are doing related to some aspect of their intrapsychic and interpersonal life. The use of "I" language in psychotherapy refers to concerns of self-disclosure and is often forbidden or cautioned to be used judiciously. Though relational psychoanalytic theory proposes a two-person psychology where the "I" and the "You" are intersecting, we are still vague about how we talk about this intersection.

The choice of pronouns can used objectively, describing aspects of separate entities, as in statements like "you do," or "you are," or "you are feeling," or "I feel," or "I am," or "you make me feel," or "we are doing," falling under what Buber terms I-It relations.

Or, alternatively, pronouns can be used subjectively, inviting reflection on how the other is experienced, linking the pronouns to subjective encounters between "I" and "You" creating a genuine "We" encounter.

When therapists use "You" statements in a declarative manner (objective use of the pronoun), it can hinder dialogue unless accompanied by the therapist's subjective experience or perceived as an invitation for further analysis by the patient rather than an absolute truth about themselves.

The objective use of the pronoun "I" can lead to self-referentiality, where the patient becomes a vessel for the therapist's projections and emotional needs. Conversely, the subjective use of "I" is contextualized within the patient's subjective experience and serves to enrich the analytic conversation.

Utilizing "We" statements can be challenging, particularly when used assumptively and declaratively. In emotionally charged situations, individuals may resort to "We" statements to diminish personal responsibility instead of acknowledging their own participation or discomfort in acknowledging the patient's contribution. In times of dyadic tension or conflict, the use of "We" should be emergent and maintain individual subjectivity while respecting the patient's unique perspective. "We" emerges when the therapist's subjective viewpoint, emotions, and experiences are shared, and the patient is encouraged to do the same. Relational "speak" means traversing to the other's side without losing oneself entirely. It is about maintaining presence on both sides of the interaction, avoiding the pitfalls of either self-absorption or complete self-negation.

In objective usage, pronouns seek to describe and name either the self or the other. In contrast, the subjective application involves delving into the experiences generated between the "I" and "You." Relational articulations aim to intertwine these pronouns into the collective "We," connecting the therapist's subjectivity directly to the patient's narrative. This shift transforms the therapeutic endeavor from a mere exploration of one's past into an interpersonal interaction where transference is experienced and worked through in direct relation to the therapist.

Relational interpretations go beyond cognitive insights by attending to the therapist's affective, experiential, and bodily involvement, emphasizing the unfolding relationship and interaction within the therapeutic dynamic. We measure the effectiveness of our articulations on how patients receive our words, on how the therapist receives the patient's response, and whether the interaction enhances analytic conversations. It is crucial to recognize that what we say is less important than how it is said, how it is received, and how it is processed between the therapist and their patient through intersubjective play.

In the unfolding of psychotherapy, we move in and out of both the objective use and subjective use of these pronouns. The only way we can measure the effectiveness of our use of them is if we have made contact with the patient and further analytic inquiry is achieved. A unique property of RPT is to create analytic conversations where the "analyst is seen less as a semidetached observer of the patient's operations and more as a full participant in interpersonal patterns they create and maintain together" (Mitchell, 1993, p. 195).

But how do we do this? What is "relational speak?" How does it differ from traditional transference interpretation language? I refer to this shift in language as a move from interpretation into a complex dialogue of working within the space of intersubjective play or as Atlas and Aron (2018) aptly term "dramatic dialogues." Premised on the belief that patients benefit not only from understanding how their past manifests in the present (transference interpretations) but also more importantly how their personal narrative is perceived, experienced, and worked through with another person (relational interpretation/articulations). A subjective language that prioritizes analyzing the relational encounter informed by the patient's intrapsychic and interpersonal configurations lived out in direct relationship to the therapist. From this relational perspective, the transformational aspect is not simply "telling" the patient *what* they are doing, healing happens when the therapist risks "being in" in the drama that is being enacted.

Thus, in the MAMAL method, less focus is on perfecting an objective *correct* interpretation. Rather, the MAMAL method practices through role-play, the development of a relational language and mindset. As languages are tricky, I forefront my effort at creating nuanced speech by suggesting that within the group consultation process, whatever words participants find to speak, we measure our effectiveness by asking (a) did the articulations expand each members' imaginations, deepen their affective states, and further understanding of repetitions? and (b) did the words/articulations advance the group members to move the therapeutic dyad into the realm of intersubjective play, a place where therapist and patient move into the space of ongoing inquiry, co-metabolizing, collaborating and enabling the capacity to "co-laborate," meaning to "labor together" (Oord, 2019, p. 153).

Though, I will now endeavor to illustrate below a shift into relational language using case studies, it's essential to acknowledge that verbalizing an experience on paper lacks the context, mood, and personalities inherent in lived subjective moments. Furthermore, our words must always be understood as second in command of how the patient hears them and how the therapist and the patient navigate the conversations that emerge. With those limitations in mind in the cases presented below, my goal is to demonstrate the nuance of advancing objective interpretive language into speaking relationally that invites patient and therapist to work within the complex space of intersubjective play.

Psychoanalyst Dr. Glen Gabbard was interviewed in *Psychology* Today by Ryan Howes (2016) where Howes asked Dr. Gabbard to describe a transference interpretation. Here is an excerpt from that interview. He begins:

A transference interpretation is often thought to be one of the most mutative interventions in psychoanalysis and psychoanalytic psychotherapy. The idea is that something from the patient's world of internal object relations is being repeated in the here-and-now interaction with the therapist, but the patient is unaware of it. The interpretation of the transference situation is designed to make something conscious that has been unconscious.

**Interviewer: What does it look like?**

A transference interpretation links three sides of a triangle. One side is the patient's transference to the therapist; a second side is the patient's experiences with current relationships outside of therapy; the third side is the patient's past relationships with parents and others. So, it might sound something like this:

"When you express your fear that I will criticize you if you speak openly here, it sounds so much like your fear of speaking forthrightly to your husband that you brought up last week and your anticipation of criticism from your dad that you brought up a few minutes ago. I'm wondering if you have retreated from your intimate relationships with men for fear that we will all put you down for having your own views on things."

**Interviewer: How does it help the client?**

Transference interpretation helps our clients by enabling them to see broad patterns of fantasies, interactions, and object relations that they had never put together before. When the same fantasy or pattern emerges in the relationship with the therapist, it is much more difficult to disown it or deny it.

**Interviewer: In your opinion, what makes transference interpretation a cool intervention?**

What makes this intervention "cool" is that it links information in the here-and-now unfolding before your eyes with the ancient past in a way that helps the patient see that the ghosts of childhood continue to haunt him or her in the present moment.

So, what is missing? Gabbard says that a "transference interpretation links three sides of a triangle. One side is the patient's transference to the therapist; a second side is the patient's experiences with current relationships outside of therapy; the third side is the patient's past relationships with parents and others" (ibid). From a relational point of view, what I see is absent in Gabbard's use of the image of a triangle is a fourth element critical to relational psychoanalytic theory. That is the subjectivity of the analyst. What Gabbard's interpretation does not demonstrate for us is his affective subjective experience with his patient. We are left wondering about his feelings as the patient's world of internal object relations is being repeated directly with him. What feelings does he experience with his patient's fear of being criticized by him? If his interpretation is correct that his patient retreats from intimacy with men for fear that she will be put down for having her own views on things, how does he experience her retreat from him? With relief? Sadness? When he interprets her fear she will be criticized by linking this to the patient's father and husband and men in general, what does it feel like for him, to have a reluctant patient in expressing herself freely toward himself? Does he wish to reassure her? Does he feel pity, anxiety, protective? Does he feel angry with her or impatient with her for her passivity? Is he paying attention to how these emotions stimulated within him are relevant to this patient's internal world and her expression of herself in her current relationships?

We just do not know. His subjectivity is not available to us nor to the patient. But what we do know is that our patients benefit not just from seeing how their past is expressed and repeated in the present and what is laboring in the unconscious (transference interpretation), but how another person (the therapist) directly experiences that past, i.e., in the here and now with the therapist. As I conjecture on possible affective experiences that may emerge within Dr. Gabbard, I can't help surmising that if the patient could have access to both his mind and his affects would increase her ability to understand not only how her past has formed her but also how in the here and now she is being experienced with Dr. Gabbard. In working directly in the here and now, a much more robust conversation deepens.

Relational interpretations seek to enlarge transference interpretations and are useful because of a fourth element, that is, the subjectivity of the analyst and the relational/interaction dimension between the two. Aron and Atlas (2021) speak to our interpretations/interventions/conversations in this way, "not only does every intervention reflect the analyst's subjectivity, but it is precisely the personal elements contained in the intervention that are most responsible for its therapeutic impact" (p. 93). Aron goes on to say (2018):

> Rather than understand transference, or any illusion, such as idealization, as simply a form of defense or as a developmental striving, Mitchell views the patient's presentation as an invitation to a specific form of interpersonal interaction, an invitation to the analyst to dance in the patient's steps, that is to enter a dramatic dialogue.
>
> (p. 55)

Thomas Szasz (1963) warns that in "psychoanalytic theory, the concept of transference [interpretation] serves as an explanatory hypothesis, whereas in the psychoanalytic situation, it serves as a defense for the analyst!" (p. 435).

When we speak of the use of the self/other relationship as a primary means toward understanding our patient, we are talking about attending to the experience the therapist has in the presence of the patient and the experience the patient has of the therapist. The shift moves us beyond formulation into how our formulations, given the data we have accumulated, are experienced, explored, and elaborated.

The following is an attempt to demonstrate a possible relational articulation using Dr. Gabbard's original transference interpretation, followed by how I might articulate my thoughts to this imaginary patient.

Gabbard's interpretation:

> When you express your fear that I will criticize you if you speak openly here, it sounds so much like your fear of speaking forthrightly to your husband that you brought up last week and your anticipation of criticism from your dad that you brought up a few minutes ago. I'm wondering if you have retreated from your intimate relationships with men for fear that we will all put you down for having your own views on things."

Barsness articulation:

> I am thinking about your fear of men and your retreat from intimacy with men for fear of being criticized. I think it is also happening here (here I am trying to connect how I see my patient and me playing out in the in-between shifting the therapeutic conversation to attending to how the past is being repeated in the here and now).
>
> Sometimes I find myself hesitant to say anything to you for fear of being critical. But when I do that, I see how I am contributing to keeping us away from closeness. Often, I catch myself wanting to "tell" you about you rather than staying in your/our experience. (*here I am acknowledging my experience and my participation in the transference/ countertransference relationship and taking greater emotional/relational risks with my patient and hopefully offering a deeper understanding of how she is experiencing and influencing her relational world*).

This relational interpretation created from the original interpretation still holds to the repetition of the past but brings it directly into how the past is being experienced in the present.

Though Gabbard's interpretation is insightful, it does not give the patient and himself the opportunity to work out her past as she is living it out directly with him. It is important to remember that it is not our explanations that are transformative. Transformation occurs when a person is met at a profoundly deep level with someone willing to risk how it feels to be in their presence.

## Case Study One

A supervisee presented the following case:

> Jean is a 60-year single, female who I have seen for a year and half. She came to therapy wanting to work through disappointments in her life- namely a failing business and multiple failed relationships. She has been married once in her thirties to man that hid a cocaine addiction from her and had been physically abusive at times. They have one young adult daughter together. She is the only living member of her immediate family. At her initial session after recounting a painful past of fractured relationships, feeling abandoned by family members and themes of powerlessness, she stated, "I still feel like I am living in trauma all of the time." She recently took 6 weeks off due to a change in her work schedule and just recently returned. At her first session she expressed ambivalence about returning. On the one hand she felt enthusiastic, on the other hand she was fearful that I did not share her enthusiasm. She tearfully asked me, "Do you really want to work with me?" I was caught off guard at the sudden turn from confident enthusiasm to fear and insecurity. In past sessions Jean has displayed similar moments of unexpected fear and anxiety about the possibility of therapy ending abruptly, leaving her feeling abandoned and unwanted. I have felt perplexed by these sudden emotional fluctuations and reflective about how fears of our relationship echo her past experiences of failed family and romantic relationships.
>
> Our work generally feels playful, engaged, and full of momentum. Then there are moments where I am left bewildered, as she spirals into self self-loathing towards her body, age and singleness, and her childlike fears. At times, these emotions leave me feeling distant and powerless, akin to witnessing self-injury and helplessness. I recognize in myself a tendency to either comfort Jean or distance myself as an outside investigator rather than being fully present. Through consultation I have begun to reflect how this pattern stems from my own childhood experiences of my father's abandonment of my family leaving me oscillating between comforting my mother in her depression or distancing myself as an outsider. This analytical, investigator stance serves as a protective barrier against confronting difficult emotions, particularly Jean's despair and feelings of being unwanted. "I seem to view both these women, the patient and my mother, through a similar lens, perceiving them as phenomenal women and perfect victims. Sometimes I want to get close, other times I want to run the other way. Or I have found awayto do both at once, where we are together yet disconnected, mutually frustrated and dissatisfied."
>
> Jean had a challenging upbringing in a conservative religious household with an absent mother, a demeaning father, and two older male

siblings who continually teased and mistreated her. She often felt alone and neglected, leading her to wonder if the chronic shame she experienced as a child was linked to her cancer diagnosis, she received at age sixteen. Jean often felt invisible, unloved, and struggled with low self-worth, hampering her ability to form loving relationships.

Her adult life has been shaped by a rare physical disability, motivating her to seek solutions as an entrepreneur and innovative business owner, a business which is currently moving into bankruptcy. Jean sought therapy with me after her previous therapist, who under the influence of drugs during a session, criticized her for her failed relationships, stating, "You're trying too hard, that's your problem, and that's why no one wants to be with you." Jean initially brushed off the behavior as "a little inappropriate," and then felt abruptly abandoned when the therapist proceeded to terminate their sessions stating he "felt embarrassed by what he had done and could not help her." For Jean this was one more experience of a failed relationship in her life.

In a more recent incident, Jean was banned from the library for damaging a book and facing what she perceived as an unjust and embarrassing fine. Refusing to pay the fine or investigate the ban further, Jean decided to no longer return to a place she once cherished. As Jean shared this story, my view of her as a victim was disrupted, prompting a realization of Jean's role in creating some of her own adversities where she becomes the victim. I sought supervision on this case to help me see what I was wrapped up in. I knew something was happening between me and Jean that I could not fully understand-both her behavior and my own.

The therapist presenting this case was hoping to break out of her over-identification with the patient, make use of the disruption that she was experiencing from seeing another side of her patient's story, and to find a way to move into a space of intersubjective play in contrast to feeling like an outside investigator. In the following I will try and demonstrate relational articulations that may place the therapist and the patient into a place of mutual inquiry of the patient's history and its repetition within the therapeutic encounter. These articulations emerge from attending to the patient's past, the therapist's past, the affective experiences, and how affect and repetition manifests itself in the therapeutic relationship.

First, I will suggest a transference interpretation that does not include the therapist's subjective experience. It might sound something like this:

> Sometimes our work feels cold and scientific. When you talk about your difficulty in finding an intimate relationship, I think you approach me and your other relationships similarly. I believe this is a way to protect yourself from being hurt by others, just as you experienced your hurt from your father.

A relational articulation might sound like this:

> In our sessions, I have noticed that I often wish to remain in an investigator role with you always attempting to unravel the cause of your hopelessness. I think I might be avoiding my feelings of despair and fully experiencing the despair that you feel by my wanting to identify and fix what seems broken. However, I have come to realize that in doing so, I am in some ways, perpetuating the narrative of your life—where you have felt objectified, abandoned, unseen, and left alone, estranged from others.

We could imagine a further elaboration to sound something like this:

> As you talk about your loneliness and inability to form intimate relationships, I have also been wondering if what I am experiencing is how you and I may be setting up our relationships in such a way that keeps us distant, cold, and scientific as a protection against being harmed once again and risking closeness.

What you see in both articulations is the use of the pronouns "I," "You," and "We." In the first interpretation they are used objectively. In the second articulation you should get more of a sense of the "I" and "You" used subjectively and a move into the space of intersubjective play. In the relational articulation the therapist has offered how she has caught herself repeating the patient's narrative by acting in a similar pattern to the patient's primary caregivers. She is offering to her patient her contribution to how she discounts the patient's feelings through scientific investigation while also inviting the patient to consider the patient's part in the repetition.

Let's now take a look at the situation where the patient has been banned by her previous therapist and by the library by first demonstrating a possible transference interpretation that does not include the therapist's felt experience. It might sound something like this:

> So, I have been thinking about your ban from the library and being banned by your therapist and about your ambivalence asking me if I want to work with you. In the case of your therapist, he banned you from seeing him again, but in the library banning you have a choice. By paying the fine of a book you damaged you would be welcomed back. So, on the one hand, in the case of your therapist you are rejected, but on the other hand, in the case of the library, you are the rejector.

A relational articulation might look something like this:

> I think there might be something similar going on here with you and me. You began your session today wondering if I am ambivalent about

working with you. My first response was to reassure you. But is it possible that on the one hand you fear I will reject you -as your therapist did, or that you will reject me like you did with the library? Despite our mutually expressed desire to continue working together, is it possible that we are reticent in our work together and always leaving a space open to leave. Perhaps, we both have only one foot in the door protecting ourselves from being rejected. Ambivalence feels safer than enduring anticipated pain.

In this articulation, the therapist holds onto the patient's storyline, recognizing recurring patterns and conveying this awareness to the patient. But at the same time, the therapist is disclosing her own thoughts and actions related to the observed patterns and her experience of them, creating a more transparent dialogue, leaving room for the patient to respond.

These articulations arise from the therapist's self-experience where the patient's narrative reverberates in the present moment. The therapist identifies defensive structures within the therapeutic relationship and communicates these insights in a way that reflects the lived experience within the session. This approach stands in contrast to interpretations that merely provide intellectual insights about the patient. Relational articulations seek to blend insights into the patient's story with the therapist's genuine felt experience. This integration allows for a more profound understanding of the patient's dynamics, fostering a richer therapeutic encounter that goes beyond a transference interpretation to encompassing a shared experiential exploration of the patient's narrative.

In these efforts to demonstrate the expression of the use of the therapist's felt experience, it is important to note that more important than the words we find to use, the key element is to ask: "Am I in touch with where these words are coming from (our affective experience of the patient) and are they embodied? Or, am I offering them in a detached way?"

**Case Two**

At the end of the session standing at the door my patient says, "I will not be here for our next session, and I think your policy of having to pay for missed sessions sucks and I won't be paying for it!" He shuts the door aggressively.

My first reaction was wow! I felt angry, controlled, misunderstood. As he knew my policy also offered make-up sessions for missed appointments, I felt reactive and the line that came to me was, "It has to be his way or the highway." I had some time to work through my emotions and saw that I had a couple of options to offer him upon his return. One, was to remind him of my policy and to expect him to pay or set up a make-up session. Two, knowing his relationship with his father, a controlling, manipulating man who was not negotiable, I could interpret his anger as a transference event and that he was treating me just as his father treated him. But as I thought about it, I became more interested in working on the experience of his past directly in the here and now of the transference, occurring in the in-between the two of us.

When he returned for his next session, it was as though he had forgotten what had happened and said nothing of our ending moments from the previous session. I was surprised and a bit miffed honestly and so finally mid-session, I said, "Are we going to talk about our last session?" "Hell ya!" he responded but continued in yet another direction. Again, I felt controlled and angry. Finally, he said, "I am not paying for last week's session, your policy sucks." I said, "Ok let's talk about it." I continued, "After you left, I felt a bit stunned and angry and the line that came to me was, it must be "your way or highway" and that I get to have no say in the matter." He cracked. And said, "That is the story of my life, it always has to be my way." By entering my own felt experience into our conversation, or we might say how the transference went "live," opened how small and controlled he felt in his father's presence. And that he often felt similarly in his relationship with me. He felt he needed to protect himself. Fearful of being controlled, he felt he had to control first. By offering my felt subjective "I" experience while remaining curious and open to his "I" experience not only moved us deeper into the hurt and anger of his past, but also to how these early object relations were repeating themselves with me and others in his relational milieu. It interrupted our repetition, expanded our conversation, moved us out of the "doer-and-done-to" enactment we were perpetuating and into a livelier space of negotiation.

## Case Three

Mark came to see me twice a week. There was not a session that went by where my eyes did not glaze over. I felt extremely bored, hopeless, and dissociative. At the beginning of each session he would ask, "So what did we talk about last session?" The groan inside me was palpable, but my standard response was, "I do not recall, and you?" He would reply, "I don't either." And off we would go both dissociating from our felt experiences. Then one day when he asked the question I said, "I have no idea, nor do you, and I am wondering if both of us feel as though there is nothing in your life that we have found is worth remembering?" He quickly agreed, interrupting our dissociative states, and we were awakened to the hopeless despair he felt as a child. A smart but ignored child. Unpopular at school. A home where no one spoke to one another. A childhood where he escaped into comic books and computers and occasionally his father's Playboy magazines scattered around the house. For months we had co-conspired to avoid the ache of his past life, when I finally expressed my felt subjective experience about what I thought "We" were doing, we connected. As I became aware in how he and I were actively recreating his past story directly with our story and truly felt the agony of his aloneness, he felt he had finally ignited an emotion in someone, and in turn, became more animated in bringing himself to me. Though we had talked *about* his story (endlessly) it was only when I finally allowed myself to *feel* his story and to be *in* the story and how awfully boring his story had become *to us* that generated an important relational shift in our work.

Stephen Mitchell viewed the patient's presentation as an invitation to a specific form of interpersonal interaction, an invitation to the analyst to dance in the patient's steps, that is, to enter into dramatic dialogues (Atlas & Aron, 2018, p. 55). With Mark, I had been sitting on the sidelines, uninterested in dancing with him. But when I acknowledged that we were both at a dance but not dancing, and offered my awkward invitation to dance, he said, "Yes." The intent of relational articulation is to move the therapeutic couple into the dance of the patient's life.

## Case Four

Paul a 37-year-old male was psychologically sophisticated with a good sense of his personal issues, quickly identifying and correctly so, himself as having an anxious and avoidant attachment style. His personal diagnosis served as a forewarning for how our work would unfold. Upon my return from a month-long sabbatical a year-and-a-half into our treatment, he announced that he would be leaving treatment to enter a treatment with someone within his insurance network. I told him that though I understood the financial incentive, that he and I both knew that there was something else at play. He agreed that this break in our fledgling attachment gave him the opportunity to detach again with someone with whom he had become attached. As the session proceeded, I asked him, "As you returned today, what did you imagine I might think or feel about your announcement?" He said, "I thought you would feel relief." I was about to reassure him that I would miss our work together, when it dawned on me that in fact, he had read me correctly, I did indeed feel some relief. So, would I tell him so? Or offer him a transference interpretation, one already swirling in my mind sounding something like:

> Given your fathers' preoccupation with himself and his disconnect within the family and your mother who did all the right things in keeping a family together but was affectively absent, leaving you to feel insecure and avoiding connection for fear of rejection and hesitant to attach, I can see why you might choose to leave, to detach from this work.

However, what I chose to say was:

> You caught me. You are correct, I am feeling some relief. It is hard to work with someone who approaches and then leaves. We have acknowledged that at times you poke at me to see if I will reject you or test me to see if I have remembered you fully. To check to see if I care, or to see if I am worthy of our trust. Sometimes I fail, sometimes I don't. Sometimes you stay, sometimes you retreat. And here we are.

We did decide to schedule one final session and the patient stated he felt relieved and a bit surprised that I would answer him directly. He said he felt validated in what he thought and knew in his own mind to be true. He also asked if I would continue to work with him until he found another therapist. I smiled and said, "Again, one foot in, one foot out." Then he smiled and said, "I understand." We ended our work—both holding a bit of sadness and gratitude. As my response was in contrast to his early attachment experiences, we could have linked his past to our present moment, but as we already knew of this, the session trended toward enjoying the genuine attachment that we had both just encountered.

Therapy is filled with a lot of talking and telling, constructing ideas, and interpreting. Our therapeutic conversations vacillate between a continuum of thinking about (I-It) and experiencing and witnessing with (I-Thou). Though transference interpretations have been considered the work horse of psychoanalysis, it is when our transference interpretations are reconsidered with the therapist's subjectivity present and the therapeutic pair risk talking *with* one another that defines what is at the heart of relational psychodynamic work. The use of the self of the therapist and working intersubjectively is the primary means of gaining access to unconscious motivations, affects, defenses, and relational blockages in the patient's life.

The "I," the "You" and the "We." Tricky. Nuanced. But you know it when it happens because you can feel it by the contact that is felt between the therapist and the patient. Buber calls this a genuine meeting or an "I-Thou" encounter. To genuinely encounter the other, we must move out of the safety of intellectualization into deeper reflection and emotion—the genesis of effective change.

Robert Grossmark (p. 89) gets at this in his important work, *The Unobtrusive Relational Analyst,* He states:

> The focus of psychoanalytic understanding is therefore shifted from interpretation of the content of the patient's world in terms of their unconscious meaning to a more all-encompassing registration of the ongoing relationship that the patient is unconsciously creating in the analytic relationship...patients do not *tell us* about these aspects of their internal world so much as *show us* in the way that they relate to and use the analytic situation and the analyst...in tuning one's analytic ear to this register of unconscious communication, the analyst must use his or her countertransference, which is, according to Joseph (1985) the 'essential tool of the analytic process'.
>
> (p. 157)

Jung (1928) said, "Even the man we think we know best...is at bottom a stranger to us. He is different. The most we can do, and the best, is to have at least some inkling of his otherness, to respect it, and to guard against the outrageous stupidity of wishing to interpret it" (pp. 220–223).

## From Affect-Metabolization-Articulation-to Intersubjective Play

When we offer our articulations through our affective experiences and the thoughts that accompany our affects, we surrender are articulations into the place of intersubjective play.

Intersubjective play is that place where both patient and therapist (two subjects) process together, co-metabolize their thoughts, emotions, and experiences in the service of deepening the life of the patient. Shifting the emphasis of the objective therapist with whom the patient projects dissociated aspects of the self onto the therapist, and the therapist interprets—intersubjectivity understands the therapeutic relationship as one of mutual influence—two subjectivities at work.

Like the sandbox or playing field of childhood, therapists and patients find themselves caught up in recreating past playbooks while simultaneously co-creating a new narrative. In the interplay of the past and the present, where the past can be re-experienced and re-formed within the unfolding story with the therapist, the patient can recover the harmed self and discover new modes of being. It's crucial to recognize that childhood play can be robust and even harmful. Therefore, the idea of play in therapy suggests that the give-and-take of successful play often emerges from hard-fought differences and conflicts into an alternative option. This option results in either recognizing the other as a contrasting partner with whom one can negotiate and/or facing the reality of a winner/loser dynamic. Successful play may imply harmony, but it also lends itself to the acceptance of failure. As Winnicott proposed (1971), it is in playing, and only in playing, that the individual, whether a child or an adult, can be creative and use the whole personality. It is only in being creative that the individual discovers the self.

This richness is compromised when the therapist is unable to bear conflict. It is common when conflict arises for the therapist to defer to what the patient wants rather than perhaps what the patient needs. In the space of intersubjective play it is vital that the therapist not surrender their thoughts and ideas too soon. This is a common practice when the patient disagrees or appears hurt or misunderstood by the therapist. The immediate default is to move away from the therapist's experience in these situations. The therapist must remember that their thoughts, their affects, and their experience were occasioned by the patient and though incomplete and requiring co-metabolization, should remain steadfast in their experience, until the patient and the therapist are able to make meaning of the experience. This may result in impasses and enactments, but when worked through, become the most meaningful aspect of the work.

## Role Play in the MAMAL Method

Role play is a common and valuable aspect of the MAMAL method, used to practice moving from *affect* to *metabolization* to *articulation* and into intersubjective play.

Once the Presenter has completed presenting the case, attention shifts away from the group assessing and commenting on either the Presenter or the patient presented. Instead, the focus turns toward attending to the affective states the patient (now considered the muse) has initiated within each group participant's own affective experience.

With the patient no longer the primary focus but rather serving as the inspiration for each participant's own affective reactions, participants begin to reflect on what affective states are being stirred up within themselves and why. They ask themselves: If this were my patient, how would I consider these affective states? How are these emotional arousals connected to the patient's historical narrative? How is the past being repeated with me, and what do I feel about that? How are these emotions, pulling up my own story and how are they connected to the patient/muse and how might I speak about this experience with the patient/muse?

This reframing encourages participants to mull over their own personal affective experience of the presenting patient, understanding that their own experience is all they have and is the most valuable contribution they can make to the Presenter and to the other participants. Adopting this stance erases the problem in role-plays where persons falsely think they can assume the experience of either the therapist or the presenting patient. When attention is focused on one's own affective experiences, their own thoughts about how this patient infects them and how they might articulate their experience, the clinical minds of all participants, including the Presenter, are enhanced.

In the role-play, participants taking on the roles of therapist or patient are inspired by the presenting patient (the Muse) but do not attempt to replicate what they believe the presenter of the case would do, nor do they try to imagine what the actual patient might say or do. Instead, the role-playing participants are encouraged to engage with their own subjective and emotional experiences, immersing themselves fully in their own unique affective states, co-creating a new and distinct dynamic. When role players attempt to mimic the actions of the presenting therapist or patient, the presenter often feels misunderstood. However, when the role-players (and all the group participants) address their affective and metabolizing processes, clinical understanding is enhanced. Furthermore, the immersion of each members own affective experience that expands  clinical understanding, will always connect, in some way, to the experiences of the presenter and the presenting patient. As Nancy McWilliams (2021) notes that when she role-plays the therapist with a particular patient, she immediately finds herself; "in the same emotional quagmire from which the presenter has been trying to get extricated" (p. 101). This reflects the power being alive to the affective responses elicited within us in response to our patient's narrative. The purpose of the role-playing exercise is to deepen each participant's insight into the therapist's self, emphasize the importance of affect, and provide practice in metabolizing and articulating experiences. The exercise fosters a space for play, engagement, and the exploration of one's affective responses. This setting discourages the tendency to focus on doing things correctly but instead promotes a deeper understanding of the therapeutic processes inherent complexity.

## Laughter

Lastly, when we play, we should laugh. Taking a page from comedians who see themselves as social commentators and truth tellers and believe that humor is the most palatable way to discuss difficult issues, humor is required of us in our work. Humor is that delicate balance of knowing your patient well enough and knowing yourself, such that you can laugh at and with each other. Humor is a bonding experience and often offers a unique perspective on the painful experiences of our lives.

I appreciate Michael Eigen's take on the therapist-patient relationship and find it the perfect coda to the words I have written to describe psychodynamic psychotherapy and a particular model of supervision to enhance the clinical process. Eigen (1988) captures our work in this eloquent way, "There was nothing for us to do (he and his patient) but keep on working with the emotional fields we generated. We were filters, channels for one another, faulty, messy, leaky, usually inadequate [and] while we were together, we were all we had" (p. 28).

And what a gift it is to be involved in this wonderful sacred space—together.

**PART SIX: LEARNING**

The Learning stage of the consultation seeks to deepen the experiential component of the consultation and grow the participants understanding of psychodynamic theory and practices. The supervisor directs this time to teach key theoretical concepts foundational to clinical practice. Though a learning period is reserved at the end of the consultation, it is important to remember that the MAMAL process is not linear. The learning process is ongoing throughout the entire process and the supervisor uses in-the-moment experiences to teach theoretical concepts. During the Learning time in the MAMAL method the supervisor guides the discussion of theory grounded and linked to the experience of the case presentation. The supervisor will often go first with their reflections and note specific moments where theory and clinical practices occurred during the group process. Again, as the MAMAL process is *not linear*, teaching moments can take place at any time during the process and should also be applied throughout the consultation process.

The primary evaluating focus is on the growth of each group member's Essential I, their use of affective attunement, their ability to metabolize their affective experiences, an increased capacity to articulate authentically, and to facilitate intersubjective play. Foundational texts for theoretical references to these clinical practices are described in this text: *Psychodynamic Supervision: A New Approach* and in the text: *Core Competencies of Relational Psychoanalysis: A Guide to Practice Study and Research*. Key elements in the *Core Competencies* text are: how we *position* ourselves (therapeutic intent and therapeutic stance); how we *reflect* (deep listening); attending to the "there and then" and "here and now" (patterning/linking); and how we *engage* (repetition/working through and courageous speech/disciplined spontaneity). These practices serve as a helpful "map" for conducting our practices while acknowledging and appreciating the intuitive organic nature of our work and are a primary structure used to teach within the MAMAL supervision method.

To further elaborate, specific attention is given to:

- establishing a clear understanding of the intent and purpose of the psychodynamic endeavor
- developing radical openness to the therapist's own self as they consider their own defensive structures and effective use of their countertransference experiences
- developing a "third ear" by learning to listen from within and to grow their understanding of the use of their "viscera" as a portal to the patient's narrative.
- working within the "there and then" and the "here and now" (repetition) and linking what happened in the past to what is happening in the present, noticing the patterns that the therapist and patient are co-creating and the unique patterns that are happening within the patient-therapist dyad

- increasing capacity to stay engaged in the inevitable conflicts and enactments that emerge within the therapeutic relationship and working them through.
- developing a relational language, demonstrating a deeper understanding of the difference between interpretation and complex dialogue, and an increased capacity to speaking authentically
- gaining a greater understanding of what analytic love means and how it essentially defines a relational work as it is defined by our practices of honesty and risk-taking, merging and emerging affectively, and being radically open and willing to work through inevitable conflicts.

Participants in a MAMAL supervision will gain greater understanding of primary psychodynamic principles such as the use of the unconscious, understanding projection and projective identification from an intersubjective view, the roles of repetition, conflict, enactment, the Third, mutual recognition, multiple self-states, and parallel process. Participants will also experience a rethinking of the role of interpretation as they practice more complex dialogue when working within the space of intersubjective play and offering their authentic presence.

It is also expected that participants will grow in their knowledge, confidence, and understanding of relational psychodynamic work as an evidenced-based treatment and know and understand that relational models are recognized by the American Psychological Association to be as effective as other evidenced-based models and are recommended to be taught as such in all psychological training programs (Norcross & Lambert, 2018; Cornelius, 2018; Shedler, 2020). Furthermore, as the MAMAL method is practiced and flourishing within the community of the *Contemporary Psychodynamic Institute*, it is hoped that when one graduates from the CPI program, through the use of the model they will have an opportunity to experience a supportive community and develop a sensitivity to the importance of collaborative work in the expansion and sustaining of their clinical practices. In working the MAMAL method, participants should also be able to articulate and execute a clear relational ethic uniquely required in working relationally (Barsness & Strawn, 2018) and apply relational psychodynamic principles in working with diverse populations.

**PART SEVEN: GROUP DYNAMICS**

The goal of the MAMAL method is to develop each therapist's mind by focusing on the participants' experiences with the patient within the safety and authenticity of the group environment. Group cohesion is achieved when each member courageously shares their affective experiences of the presenting patient (the muse) and their perceptions of how these experiences are being replicated in their own lives. These insights are offered to the group for the purpose of co-metabolization. This intimate group process aims to deepen each participant's reflective capacities and foster the courage to engage in the intersubjective space of play. It also enhances respect within the group, often leading to cohesion and a sense of ongoing community.

Participants in the MAMAL method often become an ongoing community for each other becoming an "internal chorus" (Sandra Buechler, 2008) who inspire, encourage, and guide us over our lifetime. These internalized voices provide a sense of security and help manage the challenges of our profession, offering perspective during times of clinical stress.

But there are times groups experience disruption. As the MAMAL method urges radical openness and authenticity there is no hiding and it is acknowledged that the groups themselves may also experience within-group conflict.

### Within-Group Conflict Linked to the Patient's Story

When within-group conflicts emerge the group's first task is to link the conflict to the patient being presented. Just as in individual supervision, we look to see how the patient's narrative is being replicated in relationship to the clinician. In group consults we look to see how the patient's narrative is being replicated within the group dynamic.

Parallel Process is a common phenomenon where the clinician seeking supervision unconsciously recreates with the supervisor the conflict they are experiencing with their patient. Harold Searles (1955) was the first to define parallel process stating that "processes at work currently in the relationship between the patient and the clinician are often reflected in the relationship between the therapist and the supervisor" (p. 140). In the MAMAL method, parallel process is also considered and processed when it surfaces within the group itself. It is common that the patient's story (the muse) re-appears in some form and is mirrored within the members of the group.

Parallel process is often bi-directional, meaning conflicts may be instigated by either the supervisor or the supervisee or in the case of group consultation by any member of the group and is generally unconscious, similar to enactment. When within group conflict arises, it is essential the group actively attends to the conflict, understanding within-group conflict as a useful means of gaining insight into the replications of the patient's story. The working through also furthers a deeper capacity for each group member's ability for self-reflection.

For example, toward the end of a recent group consultation, it was noted that one of the participants had been silent for most of the session. When someone in the group inquired about his silence, he reported he felt "that his contributions were being ignored and that he was angry." He further reported that he found himself "losing contact with the presentation to the point where it made no sense to him and chose to withdraw."

His response elicited an immediate response of surprise among the other group members. The participants quickly became curious of their reactions toward the colleague and issued concern for how their actions may have caused the participant to withdraw. The discussion quickly moved away from the case being presented toward the care and repair of the participant feeling ignored. The participants questioned how they had missed him and sought to repair the breach. In acting in this manner, the primary rule of maintaining an inquiring mind about parallel processes and its relationship to the patient was not followed. As the group drifted away from the case and into group process, the potential of discovering how the group experience was related to the patient and the patient/therapist dyad was compromised.

I reminded the group that their first responsibility was to explore how the group members' experience was a replication between the presenting therapist and his patient. By redirecting the conversation back toward the case, the presenting therapist began to see direct parallels occurring within himself and the group and in his work with his patient. He reported that he felt uncomfortable and annoyed with the patient's demands for more intimacy and connection (like what he was feeling with the group). He felt angry that the patient did not appreciate what he was offering (similar to what he was experiencing within the group reporting that he felt that his contributions were being ignored and that he was angry) and that because of his anger toward his patient he chose to withdraw from the patient (similar to what the therapist found himself doing with the group.

By exploring the within group parallel process, the clinician reengaged with the group, felt seen by the other participants, and became more responsive to the group. Through reengagement the therapist was able to regain focus on his and his patient's impasse. He reported feeling less annoyed with the patient's demands and increased empathy and a renewed openness toward his patient. The reset within the group fostered greater access to his patient's story and he was able to link his behavior within the group as directly related to the patient's story. He recognized he was caught in a repetition with the patient's experience of her mother, who withdrew from the patient whenever the patient sought the mother's attention and hoped for connection.

This example demonstrates the importance in group supervision of maintaining focus on group conflict as a significant window into clinical material. In examining parallel processes occurring in the group, not only was the impasse broken with the therapist and his patient, but also group dynamics were positively advanced.

As demonstrated in the case above, when working through group conflict, the distinction between group therapy and group supervision must remain clear. The goal of working within-group conflict is to restore the group to a place of trust so that they can fully participate in the development of each other's capacities for self-reflection, working with affect, metabolization and articulation. It is not to work through personal issues but to restore good relations for clinical development. A guiding question when working through group conflict is, "To what extent will our exploration restore and benefit the group in furthering their clinical skills?"

### Within Group Conflict Not Directly Linked to the Patient's Narrative

Not all tensions and conflicts that occur within the group can be resolved through the examination of the replication of what is happening with the patient. Given that we consider psychotherapy as bi-directional and that our own issues can dominate our patients, the group must also explore at times how they might be using the patient to work a conflict among themselves! In this stance we are allowing the patient's story to inform our own processes.

### Within Group Conflict Unrelated to the Patient

It would be impossible to do a thorough exploration of a case and not touch upon the wounds of the clinician, the supervisor, and members of the group. It is expected that members in a group will experience reactions, positive and negative, toward one another consciously or unconsciously that arouse one's own personal narrative. When people gather, feuds are universal, and it would be crazy making for the group to ignore the potential richness of working out within group differences/impasses/enactments. Relational enactments related specifically to group dynamics are expected to occur within the group and is not only worthy of investigation but also essential for personal and professional growth.

Therefore, the question is not whether within-group conflicts will arise; rather the question is will it be acknowledged and worked through. When this occurs the group turns in on itself to explore and imagine. In the MAMAL method, group participants are asked to have a session and use their group as the muse. When deciding to set aside case consultation time and explore their group process, the supervisor assists the group in establishing a clear time-limited frame which includes:

- recognition that the group is at an impasse most likely due to historical relational traumas and the group will explore the possible transference/countertransference interlocks that may be impeding the case consultations.
- full agreement from each member that they wish to pursue and explore the impasse.

- establish the number of sessions (no more than two) to explore the conflict.
- agree to triage at the end of the time-limited exploration to establish next steps for the group.

Once the frame has been established and the group agrees to use itself as the muse, the same principles practiced within the MAMAL method are implemented. Group members,

- are required to actively listen and attend to their own subjective affective states and how the group is impacting them.
- explore resonance and difference in their experiences of the group as they hold to an inquiring stance.
- attend to the varied affective states each are experiencing.
- connect affective states to unconscious repetitions, enactments, impasses and the avoidance of conflict.
- hold the question, "What the hell is going on here anyway?"
- experiment with how they might articulate their experience to the other.
- actively negotiate differences.

When the group is successful in using their group as the muse, a deep bonding occurs. When choosing to work through within group conflict, the distinction between group therapy and group consultation must always remain clear. The goal of working directly with within-group conflict is to restore the group to a place of trust so that they can participate fully in the development of each other's capacities for self-reflection, working with affect, metabolization, and articulation. The guiding question when working through within-group conflict is "To what extent will this exploration benefit the group and further develop their clinical skills?"

If processing the group through the lens of the muse does not result in deeper bonding but further separation, it is generally a signal that relationships in the group are fragmenting. This is due to a stirring up of unresolved personal historical, unworked material of one or more of the group members. In this case, the group could benefit from a deeper exploration of their own processes separate from case consultation. Not all tensions and conflicts that occur *within* the group can be resolved, and other therapeutic means such as individual or group psychotherapy, may be necessitated.

## References

Agassi, J. (1999). *Martin Buber on psychology and psychotherapy: Essays, letters, and dialogue*. Syracuse, NY: Estate of Martin Buber.

Anderson, R. S. (1979). Theological foundations for ministry: Selected readings for a theology of the church in ministry. T&T Clark.

Atlas, G., & Aron, L. (2018). *Dramatic dialogues*. London: Routledge.

Aron, L. (1998). A meeting of minds: The importance of mutuality in the therapeutic relationship. In *The American Journal of Psychotherapy* (Vol. 52, pp. 119–134).

Barsness, R. (2018). *Core competencies in relational psychoanalysis: A guide to practice, study, and research*. London: Routledge.

Barsness, R., & Strawn, B. (2018). Courageous speech/disciplined spontaneity. In R. Barsness (Ed.), *Core competencies in relational psychoanalysis: A guide to practice, study, and research* (pp. 179–200). London: Routledge.

Barsness, R., & Strawn, B. (2018b. Chapter 12: Relational psychoanalytic ethics: Professional, personal, theoretical, and communal. In R. Barsness (Ed.), *Core competencies in relational psychoanalysis: A guide to practice, study, and research* (pp. 220–240). London: Routledge.

Bollas, C. (1987). *Shadow of the object*. New York, NY: Columbia University Press.

Bolognini, S. (1997). Empathy and 'empathism.' *The International Journal of Psychoanalysis*, 78(2), 401–410.

Brandchaft, S. (1998). Systems of pathological accommodation and change in analysis. In S. A. Mitchell & L. Aron (Eds.), *Relational perspectives on the psychoanalytic process* (pp. 211–241). Hillsdale, NJ: Analytic Press.

Brown, W., & Strawn, S. (2012). *The physical nature of Christian life: Neuroscience, psychology & the church*. Cambridge, MA: Cambridge.

Buechler, S. (2008). The internal chorus: A perspective on the therapeutic relationship. *Psychoanalytic Dialogues*, 18(1), 1–20.

Carignani, P. (2012). The body in psychoanalysis. *British Journal of Psychotherapy*, 28(3), 288–318.

Cole, G. J. (2006). A relational perspective on therapeutic action. *Psychoanalytic Dialogues*, 16(1), 39–55.

Corbett, K. (2011). Psychoanalytic listening. *Psychoanalytic Dialogues*, 21(6), 641–656.

Cornelius, J. (2018). Chapter 2: The case for relational psychoanalysis: Exploring the scientific evidence. In R. Barsness (Ed.), *Core competencies in relational psychoanalysis: A guide to practice, study, and research* (pp. 24–42). London: Routledge.

Cozolino, L. (2006). *The neuroscience of human relationships: Attachment and the developing social brain*. New York: W.W. Norton & Company.

Cozolino, L. (2010). *The neuroscience of psychotherapy: Healing the social brain*. New York: W.W. Norton & Company.

Dimen, M. (2003). *Sexuality, intimacy and power*. New York, N.Y: Analytic Press.

Eigen, M. (1988). *The sensitive self*. Jason Aronson.

Feiner, A. (1988). Reads and misreads. *Psychoanalytic Review*, 75(5), 645–661

Fosshage, J. (2000). The meaning of touch in psychoanalysis: A time for reassessment. *Psychoanalytic Inquiry*, 20, 21–43.

Freud, S. (1958). Remembering, repeating, and working through (1914). In J. Strachey (Ed.), *The standard edition of the complete psychological works of Sigmund Freud* (Vol. 12, pp. 145–156). Hogarth Press

Gladwell, M. (2006). *The power of thinking without thinking*. New York, NY: Little, Brown & Company.

Howes, R. (2016). An interview with Dr. Glen Gabbard. Psychology Today. https://www.psychologytoday.com

Joseph, M. J. (1985). On the 'analytic third.' *The International Journal of Psycho-Analysis*, 66(1), 37–48.

Jung, C. G. (1946). *C.G. Jung letters*, volume 2, 1951–1961. London: Routledge.

Jung, C. G. (1913). *Psychological types*. (Translated by H. G. Baynes). London: Routledge & Kegan Paul. (p. 198)

Jung, C. G. (1914). *The psychology of the unconscious*. (Translated by H. G. Baynes). London: Routledge & Kegan Paul. (p. 260)

Jung, C. G. (1928). *Psychological types* (R. F. C. Hull, Trans.). Princeton University Press. (Original work published 1921)

Klein, R. H., Bernard, H. S., & Schermer, V. L. (2010). *On becoming a psychotherapist: The personal and professional journey*. New York, NY: Oxford University Press.

Knoblauch, S. (2018). Patterning and linking. In R. Barsness (Ed.), *Core competencies in relational psychoanalysis: A guide to practice, study, and research* (pp. 142–157). London: Routledge.

Levenson, E. (1982). Natchez, G. (1982). Erwin Singer 1919–1980. *Contemporary Psychoanalysis*, 18, 304–306.

Macnaughton, J. (2009). The dangerous practice of empathy. *The Art of Medicine*, 19, 40–41.

Maroda, K. (2004). *The power of countertransference: Innovations in analytic technique*. Hillsdale, NJ: The Analytic Press.

Maroda, K. (2021). *Analysts' vulnerability: Impact on theory and practice*. London: Routledge.

McWilliams, N. (2021). *Psychoanalytic supervision* (2nd ed.). Guilford Press.

Mitchell, S. (1993). *Hope and dread in psychoanalysis*. New York, NY: Basic Books.

Natchez, G. (1982). Erwin Singer 1919–1980. *Contemporary Psychoanalysis*, 18, 304–306.

Nixon, B. (2019). Personal communication.

Norcross, J., & Lambert, M. (2018). Psychotherapy relationships that work III. *Psychotherapy: Special Issue: Evidence-Based Psychotherapy Relations*, 4, 303–313.

Nussbaum, M. D. (2012). *Philosophical interventions: Reviews 1986–2011*. New York, NY: Oxford University Press.

Oord, J. (2019). *God can't: How to believe in God and love after tragedy, abuse, and other evils*. Grasmere, ID: SacraSage Press.

Richman, S. (2014). *Mended by the muse*. London: Routledge.

Schore, A. (2018). *Chapter 13: The right brain in psychoanalysis*. In R. Barsness (Ed.), Core competencies in relational psychoanalysis: A guide to practice, study, and research (pp. 241–262). London: Routledge.

Schwartz, A. (2022, May 16). The therapist remaking our love lives on TV. *New York Magazine*. https://nymag.com

Searles, H. (1955). The informational value of the supervisor's emotional experiences. *Psychiatry: Journal for the Study of Interpersonal Processes*, 18, 135–146.

Shedler, J. (2020). Chapter 3: Where is the evidence for 'evidenced-based' therapy? In M. Leuzinger-Bohleber, M. Solms, & S. E. Arnold (Eds.), *Outcome research and the future of psychoanalysis: Clinicians and researchers in dialogue* (pp. 44–56). New York, NY: Routledge.

Singer, E. (1965). *Key concepts in psychotherapy*. New York, NY: Random House.

Strawn, B., & Brown, W. (2020). *Enhancing Christian life: How extended cognition augments religious community*. InterVarsisty Press.

Szasz, T. (1963). The concept of transference. *Journal of Psychoanalysis*, 44, 432–443.

Thomas, D. (2006). Reflections on infecting the treatment. *Journal of Gay and Lesbian Psychotherapy*, 10, 39–56.

Winnicott, D. (1971). *Playing and reality*. New York, NY: Penguin.

## ADDENDUMS

### Addendum 1: Setting the MAMAL Supervision Frame

At each consultation, the MAMAL process is repeated. Even as the group becomes familiar with the method, reminding them of the process reinforces and supports the group's structure. Below is a common litany for setting the frame for the consultation period.

**Introduction**: As we come together, let's take a short pause to center ourselves. Take a mindful breath and check in with your body, mind, and spirit. Where are you? What is already being stirred in you?

A poem or a quote from a reading is most often offered to reflect upon and to further center the group.

A common reading at the Contemporary Psychodynamic Institute captured from Krista Tippets podcast *On Being,* (2016) are the words of David Whyte who says,

> One of the vulnerabilities of being visible is that when you are visible, you can be seen, and when you can be seen, you can be touched, and when you can be touched, you can be hurt. All of us have these elaborate ways of looking as if we are showing up, but not showing up and this has tremendous consequences on other people's lives. One of the dynamics you have to get over with is this idea that you can occupy a position of responsibility, that you can have a courageous conversation, without being vulnerable.

The supervisor then outlines the MAMAL process and reminds group members of the following:

**Muse:** Today, _____'s (the presenter) patient will serve as our source of inspiration. Each of us should turn our attention away from supervising ____ (the presenter) or the patient. We treat the patient as though the patient is our own by attending to our own affective experiences, actively metabolizing these experiences, and imagining how we would work our felt experiences with the patient.

**Affect:** We feel before we think. As the patient is being presented, pay close attention to your viscera, your deep affective experience of the patient. Remember, you must "feel" your patient to know your patient. Pay attention to key words within the narrative that capture your attention. Notice your intuitions, urgings, reveries, and cognitive states as they emerge. Listen to the muse with your full being, understanding that through deep affective listening, you gain access to the patient's internal and external world.

**Metabolize:** As you attend to the stirrings within you elicited by the patient's story, consider the patient's history—early object relations, issues of attachment, defensive structures, and the impact of their early formations, including peer group relations, culture, and traditions. Remember that we are all formed in relationships and harmed in relationship and repeat the problems/issues in our formation as we seek to rework them into a more vitalized life. Questions you might ask are: What is being repeated here? What historical role am I being asked to play? How am I playing that out with this patient? We also ask, "what" is being repeated and "why?" What is this experience trying to tell us?" As we metabolize, we do so not just to "explain" but more importantly to "experience" more deeply the patient's experience of themselves and others and with ourselves.

**Articulate:** We practice speaking out loud our metabolized thoughts and feelings to the patient/muse. We work at doing so with humility and courage. The practice of articulation is to expand our minds about our work and deepen our affective experience of the patient, not to arrive at a correct interpretation. Articulation assists in assessing if the articulation invites further analytic inquiry and advances the therapeutic couple into the space of intersubjective play.

**Learn:** We will conclude our session by reflecting upon what each of us has learned, clinically and theoretically. However, this process is non-linear, and the supervisor and the participants are invited to point out "in real time" any moment they experience a theoretical or clinical "aha."

## Entering the Process

- The presenter of the muse shares the case and the reason they have chosen to present this patient.
- Following the presentation, the supervisor checks in with the presenter to see if any new thoughts or feelings have emerged for them as they shared the case with the group.
- The supervisor then invites each member of the group, including themselves, to express their affective experiences of the muse.
- The supervisor then asks the group to offer their thoughts about their affective experience (Metabolization) and how they might imagine articulating those thoughts and affects to the patient.
- The practice of articulation begins with either the supervisor or a group member volunteering to practice articulating their thoughts and experience to the patient.
- Toward the end of the process, the group reflects on what they have learned. The supervisor checks in with the presenter and then with each group member, using the Learning time to identify and expand upon theoretical concepts that emerged in the consultation process.

**Note:** After the muse is presented, it is common to use role-play as an effort to further understand the affective processes occurring within the therapist in relation to the muse; to express how the therapist is connecting the dots between their own experience and how it may be related to the patient's narrative (metabolizing); and to practice articulating those thoughts.

## Reference

Tippett, K. (Host). (2016, April, 7). "Seeking Language Large Enough" [Audio podcast] *On Being.* https://onbeing.org/programs/david-whyte-seeking-language-large-enough/

## ADDENDUM 2: METABOLIZATION: MAPPING THE MIND

The patient tells their story.

First, we attune ourselves to our bodies. As we listen to our bodies, we also tune our ears to key words, phrases, movements, and the overall experience of being with the person and their story. This process involves remaining radically open to our own affective states and the affective states of the patient.
Top of Form

We wonder, "What must it feel like to be this person?"

We attune to the patient's felt experience by envisioning the primary influencers in the patient's life, spanning from in utero to the present. This shift moves us beyond simply hearing the narrative and toward developing a felt sense of being immersed in their story.

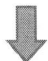

"How did this person constellate themselves given their early experiences in order to survive/thrive?"

Given the patient's experience of their story, how did they begin to construct their own sense of self in relation to their primary others (early object relations), their sociocultural experiences, traditions and contexts in which they grew up. What other influences, such as oppression, gender, sexuality, religion, politics traumas formed who they experience themselves today.

"How is the patient's past being repeated in the now?"

By delving into the patient's formative years, cultural influences, traumas, developmental milestones, and attachment patterns, we gain insight into how these factors have shaped their self-perception and interpersonal dynamics. This exploration extends to understanding how their constructed self manifests in their current relationships, including intimate connections, and how patterns from the past are replicated in their present relations as well as how it is occurring within the therapeutic relationship.

We consider how we are being pulled into the patients relational world and pay attention to how parts of our own story may be reactivated.

We pay attention to what is revived within our own story and remain cautious toward viewing it as countertransference interference. Instead, we ask ourselves, "How does my own story relate to my patient's story?" We hold to the notion that whatever triggers our own reflections or stirs something within us was sparked by the patient and therefore is most likely relevant to the patient's narrative.

We begin to imagine how we will speak our thoughts and emotions to our patients.

As we articulate our insights and observations, we strive for authenticity in conveying our understanding informed by both cognitive and affective processes. We attempt to find words that may resonate with the patient's experience while remaining open to dialogue and exploration and avoid rigid articulations that may detract from the emotional richness of the therapeutic exchange.

Upon articulation we enter the space of intersubjective play.

Intersubjective space of play is characterized by dialogue and co-metabolization where the therapist and patient engage in a dynamic exchange aimed at deepening understanding and fostering growth

Working through intersubjectively.

In the space of intersubjective play language is now being given to thoughts and experiences of the therapist and patient dyad. We expect that there will be moments of meeting and mismeetings, resonance and dissonance; where we will often catch ourselves enacting and repeating the story in much of the same way it was experienced. An unrelenting question for us to hold and to ask is, "What the hell is going on here anyway?"

It is in this particular stance that we are alerted to what is being repeated and find our way to working it through.

This stance keeps us attuned to patterns of repetition, unresolved issues, and guides us in working through these dynamics toward transformation of the past into a more vitalized self.

**And the cycle of metabolization continues.**

_____

## ADDENDUM 3: SETTING UP A RELATIONAL PSYCHODYNAMIC THERAPY (RPT)—LETTING OUR: PATIENTS KNOW HOW IT IS WE WORK

It is important when establishing a working relationship with a new patient to inform the patient of your theoretical orientation and your practices. Most new patients do not have a clear understanding of the various therapeutic models and it is important that every therapist offers to their patients their why, what, and how of their therapeutic model. It is important for a patient to know the expected outcomes of their model, the practices that will be applied to achieve those goals, what is expected of the patient themselves to maximize their therapeutic experience, and what they can expect of their therapist in their work together.

Establishing a Therapeutic Frame differs from the Informed Consent Forms that are required of us by law that inform the patient of the therapist's customary practices such as fees, frequency of visits, cancellation policies, etc. The Therapeutic Frame is what outlines the nature of our work, how we practice and therapeutic outcomes.

I will provide the reader with a glimpse into how I establish the framework in my own practice. I do not present this as a handout to the patient, and the delivery of my frame is not strictly linear. What holds significance for me is maintaining a clear understanding of my therapeutic approach and being able to organically introduce it to the patient. During the initial sessions with a patient, the dynamics of how I approach therapy and my expectations for a successful treatment gradually unfold. Toward the end of the session, I inquire if the patient has any questions about our collaboration. Often, their queries allow me to pinpoint specific moments in the session where aspects of the therapeutic process manifested.

For example, when patients arrive at my office, they press a button that alerts me that they have arrived and are in the waiting room. Recently, when I went to the waiting room to meet a new patient, he quickly asked, "Am I bothering you?" Though his question threw me off a bit, I logged it but ignored it and launched into typical first session questions, such as "What has brought you here and why me?" However, mid-session, I paused and said, "Wait a minute, your first comment when meeting me today was, 'Am I bothering you?' Is this a typical sense that you have of yourself?" He replied, "Yes."

The session then took a turn as he began to tell me about the impact of having a father who never wanted him—a father who remained physically and emotionally disengaged. He described his mother who, in response to the father's avoidance, overcompensated with excessive attention, leaving him fearful and feeling the need to keep her attention to fulfill her emotional needs.

At the end of the session, I informed him of my therapeutic position. I explained that when I caught myself missing his first comment to me, "Am I bothering you?" and then together we linked this as a repetition of his anxiety related to these two important past relationships, I was working within a relational psychodynamic perspective. This perspective, I said, seeks to link past relationships as they repeat in the here and now. This is an example of offering to the patient, organically, that is from a point within the session, the model in which I work.

Though each clinician will create their own version of their working model, I offer my own by way of example. I also wish to reiterate that unlike our Informed Consent Forms that we hand out and have our patients sign, the frame below is an internalized document of my own that evolves non-linearly. That said, I do wish my patients to have all this information and so it is common for me at the end of our first session to ask the patient if they have any questions. This is an opportune time to offer what I feel is important for the patient to know but has either not yet shown up, or they have not asked. (Note: the sample statements below are quite long to demonstrate to the reader my theory and practices. They would not be presented to the patient necessarily in this way but would be presented organically and conversationally).

### Therapeutic Frame

**Differing Modalities:** I will explain the difference between behavioral (e.g., cognitive-behavioral) and educational focused treatments (e.g., DBT, ACT) and a relational psychodynamic approach. **Sample Statement:** As you may or may not be aware there are different psychotherapeutic models, and it is important for you to know what influences me and informs my work with you. To make it simple, some therapies focus primarily on behavior and offer solutions and skills to assist you in changing a particular behavior or offer ways to think differently about a particular situation that is troubling you. Other therapies, known as depth therapies, concern themselves less about behaviors and focus on the impact on the development of the self from early childhood relationships and the cultural milieu within which one was shaped. Depth therapies pay attention to attachment issues, repressed emotions, and to how past relationships repeat in current interpersonal relations.

**Therapeutic Outcome:** I let the patient know what the key therapeutic outcomes are from a depth psychology perspective. **Sample Statement:** The goals/outcomes of treatment are discussed and respectful of each patient's hopes but generally include the following research-based outcomes: resiliency, vitalization, increased capacity to experience and manage multiple affective states and to enjoy the full range of emotion; increased access to multiple aspects of the self without shame; to comfort and soothe oneself and to be self-reflective; to accept responsibility; tolerate ambiguity and uncertainty; to be more truthful with themselves; to think more creatively and openly about one's past rather than to continue to repeat it; relief from internal constraints and rigidities that have become problematic; a more imaginative and creative mind; increased capacity to love and to work; self-efficacy; and to engage in more meaningful and redemptive relationships.

**Attending to Patients' Relational Life: Repetition.** I let the patient know that we will pay a great deal of attention to their relational life and how it tells us

something about their internal life. **Sample Statement:** As a relational psychodynamic therapist, I commit myself to paying deep attention to those relationships
in your past that shaped and formed you and still inform a good deal of how you
choose to live today. We will attend to how the past returns and replicates directly in our relationship. We will commit to working and trying to understand
the relationship that grows between us. I have found that what happened and
is happening "out there" tends to repeat itself here with me. Therefore, together
we will pay close attention to what happens between us, understanding that
working through the nuances of our relationship, you will gain deeper understanding into your own psychic structure and your interpersonal relations. Part
of our task will be to look for links between past and present.

**Attending to the Defensive Structures and the Unconscious.** I will let the
patient know that we carry unwanted emotional states within our unconscious and have created defensive barriers to protect ourselves against them.
**Sample Statement:** We will pay close attention to things that you say that
surprise you and things that you are reluctant to say. We will attend to your
dreams, as we seek to gain access to what your unconscious might be trying
to tell you about yourself. We will also pay attention to how you say things
and ways in which you wish to be perceived and understood.

**Attending to Affective States.** I will let the patient know that central to a relational approach is working with emotion. **Sample Statement:** We will focus
a good deal on your feelings. Our society privileges our mind over our affect,
and yet research tells us that we feel things before we think. I have found that
thinking often is a defense against deeply held feelings that are seeking to be
expressed and that the work of psychotherapy is to reach into the depths of
our feelings as an important pathway to healing.

**Therapeutic Expectations of Therapist and Patient.** It is important to let the
patient know what we expect of them, what they can expect of us, and an
overview of how the process of the therapy will unfold. **Sample Statement:**
Given our efforts toward a more affectively alive, deeper encounter with others, it is important that you strive to be perfectly honest with me. I invite you
to enter the therapy hour unfiltered and uncensored, to bring to me all that
comes to your mind, and to be honest in your experience of me. Our relationship differs from other social relationships in your life in that we try to come
together as unencumbered as we can and without censorship.

I will offer you the same. I will offer you what comes to my mind and what
I feel and experience with you. What I bring to you is not offered as a truth.
Rather, I offer my thoughts and experience about you, so that we can work
this experience out together.

I expect that we will encounter conflict and disagreement in our work.
We may misunderstand one another, or we may be resistant to hear what the
other is saying. I am committed to working through these conflicts and see
them as inevitable and as an important opportunity for growth.

As this is a deeply reflective work and differs from a social relationship, I
wish to be careful to attend to your thoughts and feelings and not to direct

them. For example, it is important for you to begin a session, and for me to not impinge upon what you may be thinking or what you might have experienced prior to our meeting. I trust by taking this stance that I will not set the session up in a particular way that you feel you must fulfill.

It is important that you feel free to ask me any question that you wish and to express any feeling that you may have. Our task is to work our experience together and we can only do this if you feel as though you have that freedom. If you disagree, or need clarification, or are wondering about something about me or about our work, ask and together we will try and find a way to understand what your question may hold.

**Therapeutic Fit.** It is common for us to hear friends, family members, co-workers say that they tried therapy, but it did not work, or they did not feel comfortable with the therapist. Therapist/patient fit is important for a treatment to succeed but difficult to determine, but it must be carefully considered and thought through.

I involve my patients in this consideration, letting them know it is important for them to have a good sense that I am someone with whom they could feel comfortable. In the first session, I ask them directly about their experience of me and if they feel I am someone they feel they would like to work with. I also let them know my experience of them and if I feel I can be of help to them. If either one of us expresses a tentativeness, I suggest that we take time to think about it and schedule another session to talk about it. I also suggest that if at any time during our work together they feel that we are not working well together they agree to talk with me about it first before terminating. I tell them that the reason for us talking forthrightly about this is that the shifts in our relationship may have something important for us to explore as it relates to a possible impasse in our work that we need to work through. If we are unable to work through the disconnect, I do what I can to refer them on to someone else.

It is also important for the therapist to determine if they feel comfortable and capable of working with the patient. I have always found this difficult to determine. Though in our initial meetings I may find that I am not drawn to working with a particular patient, it has never failed, that as we progress a deep regard for every patient with whom I have ever had the privilege to work, grows. I have learned that whether a patient is psychologically sophisticated and easy to work with or possesses little psychological insight, their determination to grow challenges me to find the language of my patient, identify with where they are, and grow our unique relationship.

Though I have yet to lose interest or feel a disconnect with a patient sufficient to end the treatment early, should that occur to me or any therapist, the patient needs to know what has shifted and why, and they need help transitioning to another therapist. For example, a therapist once consulted me about a female patient of hers she had been seeing for two years who recently confessed her attraction and desire for the therapist. The therapist reported feeling completely overwhelmed by the patient's attraction and promptly knew she could not continue the treatment. The therapist contacted me to work through how she would speak to the patient about her feelings and how and when to terminate.

Though I personally felt, and told the therapist, that the best treatment for her, the therapist, was to enter her own supervision and therapy and to remain working with the patient—as I believe working through scary transference/countertransference issues has remarkable potential. The therapist was adamant that she wanted to end the treatment. I then assisted her in the importance of speaking directly to the patient about her discomfort with the sexual attraction as an issue of the therapist's own and her inability to continue providing the quality of work the patient deserved. We also talked about her responsibility to help locate a new therapist for the patient.

As fit between therapist and patient is the primary determinant for success in psychotherapy (Norcross & Lambert, 2018), we must thoughtfully consider at the beginning and throughout the treatment, the quality and care—the fit—felt between the therapist and their patient.

### Reference

Norcross, J. C., & Lambert, L. (2018). Psychotherapy relationships that work III. *Psychotherapy, 55*(4), 303–315.

## ADDENDUM 4: LOCATING RELATIONAL PSYCHODYNAMIC THERAPY (RPT) HISTORICALLY MAJOR EVOLUTIONS OVER TIME IN PSYCHOANALYSIS

**Classical:** Freud, [Drive Theory] 1900 Interpretation of Dreams; 1913 Totem and Taboo, 1927 Future of an Illusion; 1939 Moses and Monotheism.

**Object Relations Kleinian:** Melanie Klein [shift from biological to psychological drives]; 1935 A Psycho-genesis of Manic-Depressive States; with Joan Riviere 1937 Love, Hate, and Reparation; 1946 Notes on some Schizoid Mechanisms.

**Object Relations/British Independent Tradition:** [shift from drives to relatedness]: 1940s Winnicott, Fairbairn: 1952 Psychoanalytic Studies of the Personality, Guntrip, Balint, Bowlby (socio-cultural context of development), Bion; Bollas: 1987 The Shadow of the Object; Winnicott (religion linked to transitional space); Fairbairn (used explicit religious language to communicate intrapsychic experience); Guntrip (Congregational minister; 1949 Psychology for Ministers and Social Workers.

Ego Psychology: Anna Freud, 1937 The Ego and the Mechanisms of Defense Erik Erikson: 1950 Childhood and Society; religion/God linked to Basic Trust; psychohistory of Luther and Gandhi Heinz Hartmann: 1958 Ego Psychology and the Problem of Adaptation conflicts in ego sphere) Rene Spitz: identified failure to thrive in infants; 1966 The First Year of Life Margaret Mahler: infant researcher; 1975 The Psychological Birth of the Human Infant (with Fred Pine and Anni Bergman).

**Interpersonal:** [focus on sociocultural and contextual factors in development] Harry Stack Sullivan 1954 The Psychiatric Interview, 1955 The Interpersonal Theory of Psychiatry; Karen Horney 1967 Feminine Psychology; 1965 Clara Thompson Interpersonal Psychoanalysis: Selected Papers of Clara Thompson; Erich Fromm; Freida Fromm-Reichmann; 1943 founded William Alanson White Institute in NYC; Sandra Buechler.

**Self Psychology:** [shift to self as construct] Heinz Kohut 1971 The Analysis of the Self, 1977 The Restoration of the Self, 1984 How Does Analysis Cure? Believed religious symbols nourished the human heart and psyche and were connected with the human need to idealize others. Thought religion could be a positive force in culture. Empathy and introspection grounded in mysticism.

**Intersubjectivity:** [sociocultural theories]: George Atwood & Robert Stolorow, 1984 Structures of Subjectivity: Explorations in Psychoanalytic Phenomenology; Donna Orange; Jessica Benjamin; Stephen Mitchell; 1985/1998 The Interpersonal World of the Infant.

**Contemporary/Relational:** [sociocultural theories, historically linked to the work of Sabina Spielrein, Sandor Ferenczi, W. R. D. Fairbairn, H. S. Sullivan] 1983 Jay Greenberg & Stephen Mitchel Object Relations in Psychoanalytic Theory; Stephen Mitchell; Lew Aron; Neil Altman; Irwin Hoffman; Jessica Benjamin; Jody Messler-Davies; Philip Bromberg; Nancy Chodorow; Karen Maroda; Adrienne Harris; Donnel Stern; Galit Atlas.

**Neuropsychoanalysis:** [brain, mind, body] Mark Solms (South Africa) 2018 "The Neurobiological Underpinnings of Psychoanalytic Theory and Therapy," Frontiers in Neuroscience; Jaak Panksepp (Estonian-American); Antonio Damasio (Portuguese-American; Oliver Sacks (British); Freud: 1895 Project for a Scientific Psychology 1999: Journal Neuropsychoanalysis first published; 2000: International Neuropsychoanalysis; Schore, A. (2018). Chapter 13: The Right Brain in Psychoanalysis. In R. Barsness (Ed.), *Core Competencies in Relational Psychoanalysis: A Guide to Practice, Study, and Research* (pp. 241–262). London, NY: Routledge. Tisdale, T., & Strawn, B. (2023). *Major Evolutions Over Time in Psychoanalysis*. This is a the reference for the above information and should be noted as a reference and not under the heading Neuropsychoanalysis Tisdale, T., & Strawn, B. (2023). Understanding the integration of psychology and theology [Conference handout]. Christian Association for Psychological Study, Louisville, KY.

**ADDENDUM 5: LOCATING RELATIONAL PSYCHODYNAMIC THERAPY (RPT) WITHIN THE HISTORICAL PSYCHOANALYTIC CANON: PSYCHOANALYSIS RE-IMAGINED**

- **Transference:** has shifted from transferring past history onto the therapist to the repetition of early childhood experiences enacted within the therapeutic relationship. The therapist is drawn into acting out scenes from the patient's history directly.
- **Countertransference:** has shifted from viewing it as interference to using the therapist's experience as potential insight into the patient's story.
- **Defensive Structures:** particularly projection, are now understood as mechanisms for survival. Projection is primarily seen as a means of communication.
- **Object Relations:** have evolved into subject relations. In relational work, there has been a move from object relations to subject relations. This relational mind acknowledges that while the patient transfers or repeats past relations, they do so onto another subject—a person with their own subjectivity, affects, and experiences, not an object. This shift necessitates a change in the therapist's neutrality, as the subject experiences the transfer directly and engages intersubjectively, with two minds working together through the transference experience.
- **Interpretations:** continue to be offered but serve as a bridge into complex relational dialogue. Emotional engagement versus neutrality highlights the difference between historical models, as the therapist attends to the psychic infections that emerge affectively.
- **The Unconscious:** is now perceived as two intersecting unconscious's, rather than only that of the patient.
- **The Conflict Model:** is viewed not only as the tripartite model of id-ego-superego but also as interpersonal conflict. The intrapsychic is worked through relationally rather than intellectually.
- **Resistance and Other Defenses:** Defensive structures are seen as manifestations of the dread of knowing what has been dissociated. The relational analyst seeks to discover where the defense is appearing within the therapeutic relationship, through interlocks and enactments. In exploring "What the hell is going on here anyway?" The analytic couple finds their way to understanding and a more vitalized life. Historically, enactments were considered acting out, but now the focus is on understanding why and breaking out of binary thinking. This process is often referred to as the Third.
- **Affect:** Historically, there was a mind-body split. In relational work, the mind-body split is seen as intertwined. The body speaks to the mind, and the mind listens to the affect. Analysis proceeds through this embodiment of the two.
- **One-Person vs. Two-Person Psychology:** Historically, the patient was perceived as an isolated individual requiring an analysis of their internalized objects. Relational theory does not discard this but emphasizes a person's

embeddedness within a social context. This directly affects treatment as the dyad engages in their own social context, patterned from the original contexts of the patient. One-person psychology focuses only on the patient's subjectivity, ignoring the analyst's subjectivity and the intersubjective exchange.

Martin Buber (1951) effectively states are situation in this way,

On this paradoxical foundation, laid with great wisdom and art, the psychotherapist now practices with skill and also with success. Until… a therapist is terrified because he begins to suspect that at least in some cases, but finally, perhaps in all, something entirely other is demanded of him. Something incompatible with the economics of his profession, dangerously threatening…What is demanded of him is …a call not to his confidently functioning security of action, but to the abyss, that is to the self of the doctor, that selfhood that is hidden under the structures erected through training and practice, that is itself encompassed by chaos, itself familiar with demons, but is graced with the humble power of wrestling and overcoming, and thus is ready to wrestle and overcome anew (Buber, 1951, p. 19).

It is my hope that this text will guide and help you in you the development of your theory and practices—but even more so, that you will never forget that it is your humanity, your dare devilishness of living boldly and authentically, humbly and fully alive—that is the ultimate healer not only for your patients—but also for you! Go live and help others to do the same.

If interested in further training and learning opportunities in Relational Psychodynamic Therapy at the Contemporary Psychodynamic Institute, please follow the link below:

www.psychodynamicinstitute.com

# Index

9781032871653